AF406285

DEDICATION

To the healthcare providers who get up daily to help and to deliver excellence to patients with voiding dysfunction. God bless you all.

Though the term "urodynamics" was not coined until 1954 by David Melvin Davis, the concept was first introduced nearly two centuries ago when Gianuzzi described the performance of manometry on dogs in 1863[1]. Over the course of time, teams of clinicians from various disciplines, engineers, physiologists, and scientists contributed to the development of modern day urodynamics, with a goal of providing objective data to assess the function of the lower urinary tract. Urodynamics has become a pivotal diagnostic tool that enhances the information upon which important therapeutic decisions are made by clinicians and patients and that also facilitates the assessment of existing treatments and the development of new options by investigators.

In 2012, the American Urological Association (AUA) and the Society for Urodynamics, Female Pelvic Medicine, and Urogenital Reconstruction (SUFU) created a joint Guideline[2] to assist clinicians in the selection and use of urodynamics in the evaluation of their patients. The guidelines, while objective and practical, do not address the inherent nuances that maximize the utility of urodynamics to guide our decisions and optimize our care of our patients.

I have had the privilege of calling Dr. Scott MacDiarmid a colleague, teacher, and friend. We have enjoyed countless hours of debate and discussion that is always stimulating and thought-provoking. Amongst many things I have learned from Dr. MacDiarmid, and perhaps the most meaningful, is his approach to the world in which we live. He is perpetually curious and constantly challenges the status quo with an inquisitive and often philosophical approach and is always pondering how to consider a topic differently, creatively, and in a more meaningful manner than the current state of the union. This book is no exception.

In this valuable work, Dr. MacDiarmid emphasizes the necessary and imperative consideration of the objective findings of the urodynamics tracings in the context of the clinical picture. The marriage of the two, infused with the experience and specialty expertise and judgment of the clinician, is eloquently and appropriately dubbed the "*art* of the lower urinary tract" by Dr. MacDiarmid. His presentation in a case-based manner is, in and of itself, artful, and this publication provides the reader with a practical approach that I believe fosters learning, critical assessment of information, and practical application of knowledge. His unique outlook should translate into optimal integration of available information and the best possible care for our patients, an aspiration that unites us all.

Kathleen C. Kobashi
Houston, TX, USA

1. Bloom DA, Wan J, Koo HP: Barometers and Bladders: A Primer on Pressures. J Urol 2000;163(3):697–704.
2. Winters JC, Dmochowski RR, Goldman HB, et al.: Adult Urodynamics: AUA/SUFU Guidelines. J Urol 2012;188(6 Suppl):2464–2472.

Contents

Introduction

The Art of Voiding Dysfunction (LUTS) is a book designed to help providers gain expertise in diagnosing and managing patients with lower urinary tract symptoms. The goal is to demonstrate how to perform the *science* of urodynamics (UDS), thereby obtaining the data that will objectively support the presumptive diagnosis, and thus direct the clinician to the appropriate treatment pathway. Although the art of medicine allows each physician to individualize treatment for the patient and the basic concepts remain the same, we will enumerate many of the nuances in the care of the patient with LUTS.

This book emphasizes the importance of a detailed history and physical examination which, combined with urodynamics and other testing, is an excellent way to establish the diagnosis and prescribe effective therapeutic pathways. Urodynamics also equips providers to better counsel their patients, set realistic expectations, and troubleshoot when necessary.

The Art of LUTS is constructed as a series of modules that bridge symptoms and signs, objective findings, diagnosis and treatment supported by literature-based guidelines, expert opinion, and personal experience. The unique modular approach extends beyond the typical

This book emphasizes the importance of a detailed history and physical examination which, combined with urodynamics and other testing, is an excellent way to establish the diagnosis and prescribe effective therapeutic pathways.

didactic discussion by suggesting treatment pathways which mimic situations in clinical practice. Pathways are efficient, they keep patients informed, and they can improve patient adherence and outcomes. With a step-by-step guide, often advancing from more conservative to invasive therapies, patients naturally find the treatment that is best for them based on an accurately diagnosed voiding disorder.

The book is written for general urologists, gynecologists, advanced practice providers, urodynamic nurses, and those fellowship trained or sub-specialized in voiding dysfunction. We hope to encourage providers to enjoy their journey delivering excellent care to this often challenging population of patients.

We are excited to present to you *The Art of LUTS* and hope that it benefits you and your practice. We are grateful to Laborie for sponsoring this endeavor; without them, the project would never have materialized.

CHAPTER 1

Guidelines vs. Expert Opinion - A Hybrid Approach

The American Urological Association (AUA) and Society of Urodynamics, Female Pelvic Medicine and Urogenital Reconstruction (SUFU) have guidelines regarding the effective diagnosis and management of patients with lower urinary tract disorders, including female stress urinary incontinence, incontinence after prostate treatment, benign prostatic hyperplasia, overactive bladder, interstitial cystitis and bladder pain syndrome, neurogenic lower urinary tract dysfunction, and adult urodynamics.[1-9] Combined with those endorsed by the International Consultation on Incontinence, the European Association of Urology, the International Continence Society, and others, guidelines play an important role in directing literature-based practice.

Guidelines represent a detailed analysis of the literature in which relevant data is extracted and its quality is assessed. Determination of evidence strength is categorized, and directive and non-directive statements are made according to the body of evidence grade, level of certainty, magnitude of benefit or risk/burden, and the Panel's judgment. In situations where gaps in the evidence exist, the guideline panel members provide guidance in the form of clinical principles or expert opinion. Each guideline's usefulness and impact are dependent on the quality of the data reviewed.

A shortcoming of the LUTS guidelines is the paucity of objective data. Many trials have small sample size, and there is patient heterogeneity across various studies. The availability of multicenter, randomized, placebo-controlled trials is limited, and long-term data is lacking. Consequently, the guidelines contain many non-directive statements, expert opinions, and the word "optional," all potentially lessening their clinical applicability. Unlike other urologic disorders like carcinoma of the prostate, literature-based diagnostic and treatment pathways tend to be less available for LUTS.

Guidelines commonly reference the "index patient." But, in clinical practice, patients are often more complex, which makes the index patient recommendations less applicable to them. We believe that an inherent bias for many clinicians to apply index guidelines to more complicated cases may affect the diagnosis and treatment pathway and therapeutic outcomes for individual patients.

The AUA adult urodynamic guidelines are similarly hampered by a lack of data. There are few well designed studies evaluating the study's ability to recommend treatment, predict outcomes, and counsel patients regarding individualized benefits and risks. In the absence of supportive data, the guideline statements that recommend their conservative use may negatively impact the care pathway in select patients. These recommendations also do not address the subtleties or the art of the study conclusions and fall short on directing how to apply urodynamics to individual patients in the clinical situation. As it is not their primary objective, the guidelines do not make firm recommendations for "Accurate Diagnosis to Treatment Pathways" which is one of the objectives of this voiding dysfunction modular series.

The recent emphasis on guidelines has also limited the opportunity to learn from clinicians who have expertise and experience in treating patients with voiding dysfunction. Many clinicians are yearning for more "how do you treat medicine" from experts who are skilled and experienced.

In *The Art of LUTS,* we recommend and present a hybrid approach that combines guidelines with expert opinion in order to improve the focus on the best way to deliver excellent care to patients with lower urinary tract symptoms.

CHAPTER 2

Urodynamics – The Current State of the Union

Urodynamics is a functional assessment that provides pathophysiologic explanations for symptoms and/or dysfunction of the lower and upper urinary tracts. It was first coined in 1954 by David Melvin Davis and published in the Journal of Urology in 1962.[10–11] In 1985, Jacques Susset described urodynamics as the "medical science concerned with the physiology and pathophysiology of urine transport from the kidneys to the bladder as well as its storage and evacuation."[12]

The authors view urodynamics as an art as well as a science. We believe that the art of urodynamics is the application of the objective findings of a well-executed study to the individual patient, taking into consideration subtleties that may be clinically relevant. Excellent patient care is driven one patient at a time, and the UDS study plays a vital role in this endeavor.

> Provider experience, knowledge, and skill plus urodynamics are better than provider talents alone when it comes to managing many of the patients with voiding dysfunction.

Urodynamics consists of a number of tests, and, when combined with the history and physical examination, radiologic studies, and endoscopy, it is an essential part of our diagnostic armamentarium. Based on individual training, experience, and interest, its utilization in clinical practice varies. It's often underutilized by those who are less interested or question its clinical value.

Urodynamic studies are many times poorly performed or incomplete. In spite of available training, it is challenging to find expert urodynamic nurses or technicians dedicated to ensuring adequate test quality. A high-quality study is necessary to maximize its clinical usefulness.

Although there are many who underscore the value of urodynamics, the reasoning seems faulted. Some say the test is invasive, but urologists routinely instrument the lower urinary tract. Others are concerned about cost, but the utility of a proper diagnosis is priceless. References in the literature demonstrate that urodynamics does not predict therapeutic outcome, but empiricism in diagnosis and therapy is not as accurate in making therapeutic decisions as objective data.

The most common argument against urodynamics is that performing the study does not change the management of patients with voiding dysfunction. However, in a tertiary complex voiding dysfunction clinic, properly performed urodynamics is instrumental in recommending treatment. The goal of this Diagnosis to Treatment Pathway Modular Series is to educate and help narrow the gap between these two opposing viewpoints. It's natural to justify one's own behavior, and we recommend an open mind when reading the modules.

How I Evaluate Lower Urinary Tract Dysfunction

For years, I've wanted to write *The Art of LUTS* and was excited when given the opportunity to do so. During this journey, my friend David Staskin, MD, during discussions and with some editing kept me in my lane. Having trained under a number of mentors all approaching patients differently, I wanted to share with you my experience and how I evaluate patients with lower urinary tract dysfunction.

Initially, I do an in-depth history and physical examination that is informative but efficient in gaining the information needed. I do not spend much time on personal chit chat or aspects of the voiding dysfunction history that are less relevant. I'm liberal in recommending urodynamics and perform video studies in nearly all cases. I don't hesitate to perform cystoscopy and, many times, the visual anatomy combined with the functional study is beneficial.

I consider four primary factors when evaluating the LUTS patient (Figure 3.1). I consider patient features, how well the bladder stores, how incompetent the outlet is, and evaluate voiding efficiency in all. And I use the history, physical, often urodynamics, and sometimes cystoscopy to analyze each one of these primary factors.

Figure 3.1 Primary factors to consider in the LUTS patient
Patient features
How well the bladder stores
How incompetent is the outlet
Evaluate voiding efficiency

Patient features

First and foremost, it's important to identify which symptom(s) is most severe and bothersome to the patient. Is it flooding enuresis, overactive bladder, stress urinary incontinence, a reduced urinary flow, or others? Identifying the main symptom(s) not only shines the light on the problem but also helps direct work up and treatment.

In most cases, symptoms take precedent over objective findings that may be demonstrated during urodynamics. For example, a patient with urgency urinary incontinence (UUI) who soaks six pads per day has severe bladder overactivity even if their filling cystometry is not that impressive. The importance of correlating these divergent findings is critical to an accurate diagnosis.

A second feature to identify is the presence of any underlying condition that may be causing the urinary symptoms. Neurogenic (CVA, Parkinsons, multiple sclerosis, spinal cord trauma), fluid balance conditions (uncontrolled diabetes, peripheral edema, sleep apnea), and other medical conditions can exacerbate voiding complaints, and treating the primary cause first is appropriate. These causal factors and how they may affect therapeutic outcome should be discussed. For instance, overactive bladder symptoms secondary to a stroke are likely to persist following an anti-incontinence operation (sling) in a woman with mixed incontinence.

Another feature deserving discussion is the presence of medical co-morbidities, especially the patient's functional and cognitive status for toileting. It's more difficult to help patients who are functionally or cognitively impaired. Treatment recommendations and expectations should be modified.

Finally, patient goals and expectations are germane to any diagnostic to treatment pathway discussion. Identifying what's most important and bothersome to the patient is vital. Offering surgery for well tolerated pelvic organ prolapse when recurrent urinary tract infections is the primary concern is not in the patient's best interest.

How well does the bladder store?

When evaluating the bladder's ability to store, I'm referring to the detrusor's filling capability independent of urethral competence. Bladder storage function can be assessed by the history, the voiding diary, and by filling cystometry. Measuring and correlating all three provides the most comprehensive assessment of the bladder storage disorder.

For example, a patient who soaks multiple pads daily due to urgency urinary incontinence has a more severe storage disorder than one who manages their UUI with a single liner. A diary recording voided volumes of 100–150 mL every 30–40 minutes represents a worse problem than one demonstrating voiding every two hours with a functional capacity of 400 mL. The presence of unfavorable storage characteristics during cystometry such as high pressure detrusor overactivity or loss of bladder compliance is more severe than a bladder with only a mildly abnormal cystometrogram.

> Bladder storage function can be assessed by the history, the voiding diary, and by filling cystometry. Measuring and correlating all three provides the most comprehensive assessment of the bladder storage disorder.

The more one listens to and evaluates female patients with mixed stress and urgency incontinence, it's often apparent that the overactive bladder is the primary problem, and recognizing its severity is clinically relevant. This information is not appreciated from an electronic medical record only stating, for example, mixed incontinence and frequency, and then copied and pasted forward as the decision-making historical account.

How incompetent is the outlet?

The assessment of bladder neck and urethral function in maintaining continence is important in patients with stress urinary incontinence (SUI). "How incompetent is the outlet" can be determined by the history, physical, and urodynamics. Using and correlating all three provides the best assessment of urethral competence.

A historical account of the severity of SUI should be documented. Leaking a few drops only while playing tennis is less severe than significant leakage with coughing, bending, walking, and with most activities, requiring multiple pads daily.

The pelvic examination in a woman with stress incontinence evaluates severity of leakage and the degree of urethral hypermobility. A hypermobile urethra that leaks minimally with a deep cough is different from one that wets your lab coat during a gentle Valsalva. A fixed urethra is not a hypermobile one in the same patient with SUI. A fixed scarred short urethra that leaks with gravity is a more complicated presentation than a normal appearing immobile one that requires a significant cough to demonstrate its mild incompetence.

Urodynamics also assesses the degree of urethral hypermobility and urethral function. The leak point pressure (LPP) has become the standard in evaluating urethral competence and identifying those with intrinsic sphincter deficiency (ISD).

A LPP of 20 cmH_2O represents a more incompetent outlet than a LPP of 140 in the same patient with SUI. Coughing repetitively and finally leaking a few drops at 60 cmH_2O is less severe than high volume incontinence easily produced at the same pressure. The degree of hypermobility can be viewed during video-urodynamics with the patient in the sitting or standing position. A rectangular-shaped incompetent bladder neck visualized fluoroscopically is consistent with ISD.

The evaluation of urethral function in men is similar. The severity of stress incontinence can be judged by the history, physical, and urodynamics.

The history provides an excellent account of urine loss and how it relates to activity and pad count. Requiring two damp pads to accommodate an active lifestyle is mild compared to soaking several Depends® daily. Some men with severe SUI never void because of their high volume incontinence which often occurs without awareness.

During physical examination, a standing positive cough test leaking a small amount with vigorous coughing is not the same as leaking continuously with gravity. Noticing a small urine stain on a patient's pad several hours old is not the same as the presence of a heavily soaked Depends® recently changed by the patient.

Measurement of the LPP is also an important part of the male SUI evaluation. Although less is understood regarding its clinical relevance, most experts would agree that leaking a few drops with a LPP of 140 cmH_2O represents a more competent outlet than one that leaks a large amount with a LPP of 30 cmH_2O. Such LPP findings may influence treatment recommendations.

Evaluation of voiding efficiency

Evaluating voiding efficiency is important in the majority of patients with voiding dysfunction. How well the bladder contracts in a coordinated fashion, how well the urethral sphincter relaxes, and whether the urethra is unobstructed dictates the efficiency of voiding and the bladder's ability to empty.

Voiding efficiency can be evaluated by the history, physical, uroflowmetry, the post-void residual (PVR), and urodynamics. Cystoscopy plays a role in select patients, especially in men. A combined approach represents the most thorough assessment.

First and foremost, listen and record what the patient says regarding their flow. A reported good or reasonable flow is different from one that is slow, stops and starts, or is associated with hesitancy and straining.

On physical exam, the presence of a large cystocele or one that hinges over a less mobile urethra could upset voiding efficiency. In those having had a previous bladder neck suspension, the presence of an overcorrection shelf visualized as hyper-elevation of the urethra-vesical angle may be a sign of obstruction.

During uroflowmetry, the flow rate and pattern help assess voiding efficiency. A maximum urinary flow rate (Qmax) of 10–12 mL/sec is different from a Qmax of 20 ml/sec in the same patient reporting flow symptoms. A long, prolonged, and reduced flow pattern is not a mildly depressed one or a normal bell-shaped curve. A spiking pattern secondary to straining or from intermittent dyssynergia is important to identify.

Determination of the post-void residual urine volume is important. Although it does not diagnose the presence of obstruction, it does determine the emptying capability of the bladder. A PVR of less than 50 mL is different from a PVR of 185 mL or 412 mL in the same voiding dysfunction patient. A mildly elevated residual may be clinically relevant in select patients.

Pressure flow is the urodynamic gold standard in identifying the presence of poor bladder contractility and bladder outlet obstruction (BOO) in patients with flow symptoms. A maximum detrusor pressure, $P_{det}max$, of 10, 60, and 100 cmH_2O has different implications in the same symptomatic patient. A fleeting contraction of 35 cmH_2O will not empty as well as

Voiding efficiency can be evaluated by the history, physical, uroflowmetry, the post-void residual (PVR), and urodynamics. Cystoscopy plays a role in select patients, especially in men. A combined approach represents the most thorough assessment.

a prolonged well sustained contraction generating the same pressure. And the corresponding flow rate should be interpreted to effectively evaluate voiding efficiency.

Electromyography (EMG) identifies the presence of urethral sphincter and pelvic floor dyssynergia. Deciding when increased EMG activity is clinically relevant often takes experience. Fluoroscopy is helpful in identifying the site of bladder outlet obstruction and any secondary chronic bladder changes.

Cystoscopy completes the voiding evaluation in many men and women with urinary flow symptoms. The presence of anatomic abnormalities, and, to some degree their relative severity, may be identified.

A difference of philosophy

Surprisingly easy to learn and efficient to deliver, I have found my approach to the LUTS patient to be beneficial and unchanging.

It's enjoyable looking at the various pieces of the puzzle in each of the four primary factors and how they support or refute one another. Then the "art" of pulling the observations from each, blending them into a final diagnosis and clinical conclusion, and selecting a treatment pathway is effective and rewarding.

As we present each individual diagnosis to treatment pathway module, we recognize the differences in how clinicians practice. Some are more aggressive in recommending invasive therapies, with or without much diagnostic assessment. Others take a more conservative and devil's advocate approach, often placing invasive treatments further along in the treatment pathway. The differences in treatment philosophy are interesting, is reality, and will and should continue since both approaches can be effective.

In our diagnosis to treatment pathway modular series, we will share with you our approach. We anticipate agreement, disagreement, and friendly criticism from others. But in the end, a healthy discussion highlighting the art of voiding dysfunction and achieving good therapeutic outcomes is a goal that we all can agree upon.

Performing Great Urodynamics

For those who manage patients with voiding dysfunction, they should excel in performing and interpreting urodynamic studies. Urodynamics is not a difficult set of tests, but it does demand a certain level of precision in order to optimize its usefulness.

Let us provide a few overarching principles that will help you perform great urodynamics in clinical practice.

Find a Brenda

It's important to find a dedicated and talented person to do the studies. Relying on an inadequately trained, inexperienced, or less interested employee will likely jeopardize quality. The number of times we have witnessed an unsatisfactory test in our referral practice is noteworthy.

We recommend for you to find a "Brenda" to perform urodynamics. Brenda has been my urodynamics nurse for the majority of my career and is an expert. Her attention to detail and detective style pursuit of defining the patient's bladder dysfunction is second to none. Brenda's lab is her own domain, and she has the freedom to manage it accordingly. She provides input regarding scheduling, knowing that some patients take longer than others.

In finding a "Brenda," concentrate your efforts on a person who enjoys urinary incontinence as well as the technical and personal aspects of the study. Keep in mind that they spend a lot of time alone with patients and have less opportunity to interact with other staff. Urodynamic technicians need basic nursing skills in order to manage vasovagal or other patient complaints occurring during the study. Spending the necessary time and resources to ensure that they are well trained is critical. A weekend course is a good start, but it will not produce an expert. Often physician input is necessary in order to teach the skill.

Take your time

Take your time performing urodynamics. In the midst of medicine's hectic pace, slow down and take time with patients explaining, instructing, encouraging, and, when needed, repeating aspects of the study to ensure its accuracy.

A careful explanation and calming words go a long way in making the test as pleasant and natural as possible. A controlled, less stressful environment improves patient satisfaction and gives staff time to focus on doing good studies while being sensitive to patient needs. The slower pace also fosters long-term job satisfaction and less staff turnover.

Our center performs four video-urodynamic studies daily. This affords Brenda the necessary time with each patient, some of whom are frail or have limited mobility. Just getting the patient undressed and dressed can be time-consuming. The few extra moments give Brenda time to document and to get ready for the next patient.

A recent quote from Brenda reads:

"Performing urodynamics is my passion. The patients I work with are struggling with embarrassing incontinence, retention, and voiding dysfunction. Usually by the time they see me, they have been suffering with these issues for some time, and their quality of life has been affected. Many of them are apprehensive about having the study, and the test requires patience, empathy, and coaching from me to proceed and to get the best study possible. It is such a privilege and joy to take care of and to serve my patients."

I pause, thinking how wonderful Brenda is and how she positively impacts our practice. Brenda, thank you for loving on our patients. Thank you for being you. Cheers!

Answer the clinical questions

Beyond performing an accurate test, answering the clinical questions being asked is the study's primary goal. Determining how well the bladder stores, how incompetent is the outlet, and how efficient is the patient's voiding should be answered, since the patient's treatment pathway depends on it. Whether the patient is considering a sling for mixed urinary incontinence or a transurethral resection of the prostate for poor bladder emptying, answering these clinical questions often has therapeutic relevance.

During the study, it's important to try to duplicate the patient's symptoms in order to identify the underlying bladder dysfunction. Don't hesitate to refill the bladder and to reevaluate when necessary. Urodynamics is not just a bladder, urethra, and a test but an important diagnostic exercise.

> Urodynamics is not just a bladder, urethra, and a test but an important diagnostic exercise.

Two-way communication

Good two-way communication between the urodynamics staff and provider is part of doing great urodynamics. The patient's history and physical examination should be reviewed by the technician prior to beginning the study. Brenda yellow highlights the most relevant aspects of my clinical evaluation and understands the clinical question being asked. It also helps her to look out for any subtleties during the study that might be important.

For example, the prolapse patient with an elevated PVR needs a voiding study with and without the prolapse reduced in order to predict whether or not the bladder will empty well postoperatively. The man with mild post-prostatectomy incontinence may require his urethral catheter removed to check for LPP's using the rectal line if he does not leak with the catheter in situ.

Effective communication travels in both directions. In Brenda's nurse impression, she documents any observations that may be relevant. Her words help convert an otherwise robotic narrative into the clinical face of the patient. For instance, she confirms whether a void was voluntary or involuntary, or whether or not it was representative of the patient's normal. She reports when a patient who is able to suppress an overactive detrusor contraction during cystometry admits that they would have leaked during the same event in public. A small radiographic shadow next to the urethra that might represent an undiagnosed diverticulum is circled and narrated.

Interpret urodynamics during the visit

I interpret and dictate urodynamics only during the patient's return visit to discuss the results. This allows me to review my clinical findings and impression prior to reading the study. If needed, I can ask the patient further questions that may be relevant. Reading the study as a separate document without knowing the patient's clinical presentation is less meaningful and should be discouraged.

Urodynamics template

I have included a urodynamics template (Figure 4.1 and Figure 4.2) with its descriptive text that you may find useful. Designing a personalized template that best fits you and your practice is a beneficial exercise.

Figure 4.1: UDS template – Page 1

Urodynamics:

Patient name:	**Patient ID:**	**Ordering physician:**
Date of birth:	**Date:**	**Supervising physician:**

Study indication:

The procedure's risks and benefits were discussed with the patient.

Pre-uroflow and catheterization:

Voided _____ ml with a Qmax of _____ ml/s.
(Voiding pattern: normal/obstructed/straining/box-like)

The patient did not void/arrived with a foley catheter.

A 14 Fr straight catheter was inserted and the volume obtained was _____ ml.

Comment: ____

Cystometrogram:

The bladder was filled with sterile water/contrast at a rate of 50 ml/min.

MCC _____ ml. (full//leaked/safe volume/pain).
Vol of first sensation of filling _____ ml, normal desire to void _____ ml, strong desire to void _____ ml, felt urgency _____ ml.
(Sensation was normal/increased/decreased/no sensation/reproduced pain: baseline pain score_____, pain at MCC _____)

The detrusor was stable/overactive.
First contraction occurred at _____ ml and P_{det} _____ cm H_2O. Max overactive P_{det} was _____ cm H_2O at _____ ml.
(Urgency/no urgency/leaked/did not leak. Vol loss: mild/moderate/severe)
(Low pressure/high pressure/recurrent/stepping/sine wave/triggered by cough/Valsalva)

The bladder compliance was normal/abnormal. (End filling pressure _____ cmH_2O)

Neurogenic: Voided by reflex detrusor contractions. DLPP _____ cmH_2O. Voided vol ___ ml, PVR ___ ml. (well/not well sustained)

Comment: ____

Figure 4.2: UDS template – Page 2 and 3

Leak point pressure:

LPP's were assessed with the patient sitting/standing and by x-ray/direct visualization/patient reporting.

The VLPP/CLPP at _____ ml was _____ cmH$_2$0. The volume loss was mild/moderate/severe.
The VLPP/CLPP at _____ ml was _____ cmH$_2$0. The volume loss was mild/moderate/severe.
The VLPP/CLPP at _____ ml was _____ cmH$_2$0. The volume loss was mild/moderate/severe.
The VLPP/CLPP at _____ ml was _____ cmH$_2$0. The volume loss was mild/moderate/severe.
The patient did/did not leak with the cystocele reduced.
The lowest LPP with cystocele reduced was _____ cmH$_2$0 at _____ ml.

The patient did not leak. The max P$_{abd}$ generated was _____ cmH$_2$0.

Comment: ____

Pressure flow study:

The patient did/did not generate a voluntary detrusor contraction.

Void vol _____ ml. Qmax _____ ml/s.
MaxP$_{det}$ _____ cmH$_2$O. P$_{det}$ at Qmax _____ cmH$_2$0.
(well sustained/reasonably well sustained/not well sustained/voided with abdominal straining/by an involuntary detrusor contraction)

PVR _____ ml. (double void PVR: _____ ml).

Comment: ____

Electromyogram:

EMG activity was measured by surface electrodes.
EMG activity normal/abnormal
EMG activity decreased/increased/remained the same during voiding.
(Increased EMG during voiding due to poor relaxation of the urethral sphincter/external sphincter dyssynergia/straining/artifact)

Comment: ____

Urethral pressure profile:

Max UPP _____ cmH$_2$O. Functional urethral length _____ cm.

Comment: ____

Fluoroscopy and VCUG:

During a cough/Valsalva the bladder neck descended approximately 1 cm or less/2 cm/more than 2 cm/ _____ cm
Bladder contour was normal/trabeculated/Christmas-tree shaped/diverticulum/cystocele/reflux (right/left/bilateral).
Size of cystocele: small/moderate/large.
During voiding: bladder neck dyssynergia/external sphincter dyssynergia/urethral diverticulum/spinning-top deformity/other:

Comment: ____

Medications given: _________________________ Teaching: _________________________

UDS summary:

Assessment:

Physician: _________________________________ Date: _________________________

Urodynamics (descriptive text)

Study indication

The indication/diagnosis for doing the study is noted.

Pre-uroflow and catheterization

The patient is asked to arrive with and to void with a comfortably full bladder. The uroflowmetry is recorded. A catheter is inserted and the PVR is measured. The voiding pattern may be documented.

Any difficulty or pain associated with insertion of the urodynamic catheter is noted.

Cystometrogram

Four primary parameters are evaluated during the filling cystometrogram, i.e., the maximum cystometric capacity, bladder sensation, detrusor activity, and bladder compliance.

The maximum cystometric capacity is measured and it's noted whether the capacity was limited by bladder fullness, pain, urinary incontinence, or a safe maximum volume was achieved. For those who report pain during the study, a rough estimate of the baseline pain score from 0–10 and the score at MCC is useful.

Bladder sensation is reported by a number of descriptors in the template. The volumes at which the patient reports first sensation, a normal desire to void, a strong desire to void, and urgency are recorded.

Detrusor stability vs. the presence of detrusor overactivity is reported. The overactive detrusor is further characterized by a number of descriptors in the template.

Bladder compliance vs. noncompliance is noted, including the end filling pressure.

In spinal cord injured patients who void by reflex detrusor contractions, the detrusor leak point pressure is measured. The volume voided, the estimated PVR, and whether the contraction is well sustained or not well sustained is recorded.

Leak point pressure

Valsalva and cough leak point pressures are recorded as well as the volume at which they are measured. The volume loss is noted. The leak point pressure with and without the prolapse reduced is recorded.

If the patient did not leak, the maximum abdominal pressure generated is noted.

Pressure flow study

The pressure flow analysis is recorded. It's noted whether or not the patient voided with abdominal straining or by an overactive detrusor contraction. The PVR is measured. If the patient does not empty well, they are instructed to double void in private, and a second PVR is estimated.

Electromyogram

The EMG activity is recorded as noted in the template.

Urethral pressure profile

The maximum urethral closure pressure and the functional urethral length are measured.

Fluoroscopy and voiding cystourethrogram (VCUG)

A narrative with descriptors is included in the template.

It's noted if a medication (such as antibiotic) was given at the end of the study, and whether or not teaching such as behavioral therapy was prescribed.

UDS summary

The pertinent urodynamic findings are summarized in a short paragraph. In addition, any nuances are highlighted so the physician can better envision the study results.

For example:

The patient was nervous and had difficulty voiding in the lab setting.

The patient did not leak during detrusor overactivity, but said that she normally would have if she was out in public.

The patient reported that her flow during the study was better than/worse than her usual.

The patient was encouraged not to strain during voiding.

There was a lot of subtraction artifact during the study.

The EMG was not recording well during the study, etc.

Functional Anatomy of the Lower Urinary Tract

A basic understanding of the functional anatomy and innervation of the lower urinary tract is germane when managing patients with lower urinary tract dysfunction.

Bladder storage depends on passive filling of a relaxed detrusor muscle and a closed urethral sphincter mechanism. Voiding is achieved by a coordinated and well sustained detrusor contraction in conjunction with relaxation of the urethra and bladder neck.

The bladder is a distensible, muscular organ composed of an interlacing network of smooth muscle designed for bladder storage and emptying. Its urothelium, lined by umbrella cells, reduces its permeability and is the first line of defense against urinary pathogens. Richly innervated by afferent nerve fibers, the urothelium releases a number of neurotransmitters which influence sensory nerve activity and alter contractile function.

In females, the urethral sphincteric mechanism consists of the proximal two thirds of the urethra blending imperceptibly with the bladder outlet. The wall is comprised of an outer sleeve of slow-twitch striated muscle, the rhabdosphincter, which produces passive urinary continence, a middle layer of smooth muscle, and an inner seal of mucosa and submucosa.

Adjacent to the rhabdosphincter lies the periurethral striated muscle of the pelvic floor, which is capable of stopping and starting the urinary stream, and maintaining continence by reflexively contracting during Valsalva maneuvers. The endopelvic fascia composed of ligaments and the levator ani muscle group supports the pelvic organs. The pelvic floor is a natural backboard to compress the urethra against during increases in intraabdominal pressure.

With the intra-abdominal position of the bladder neck and proximal urethra, increases in abdominal pressure get transmitted equally to them, helping to maintain continence. Stabilization and attachment of the mid-urethra to the symphysis pubis provides additional support.

In males, the urethral sphincteric mechanism is composed of the proximal bladder neck and the distal urethral sphincter located at the apex of the prostate. More powerful than their female counterpart, both provide passive continence. Voluntary control of the distal sphincter stops and starts urinary flow, and the prostate gland further increases bladder outlet resistance.

Control of the lower urinary tract is mediated by the peripheral and central nervous system. Three sets of peripheral nerves innervate the vesicourethral unit. The sacral parasympathetic pelvic plexus (S2–S4) primarily innervate the detrusor muscle, and are responsible for bladder contraction and micturition. The thoracolumbar sympathetic hypogastric nerve (T10–L2) inhibits detrusor activity and increases contraction of the urethral sphincter, both important for bladder storage. Voluntary control of the pelvic floor and urethral sphincter arise from the somatic pudendal nerve (S2–S4). Sensations of bladder filling or stretch are primarily mediated through the parasympathetic pelvic plexus.

The balloon model

The *balloon model* is a simple and practical approach that can help providers conceptualize urinary incontinence and voiding symptoms in men and women (Figure 5.1). No matter how complicated or unclear the presentation is, the underlying dysfunction always reverts to the balloon. This simplification of urinary complaints assists in prescribing treatment pathways.

From a patient's perspective and understanding, the balloon model helps simplify their symptoms. It rationalizes why urodynamic tests are ordered, and enables providers to clearly explain the voiding dysfunction problem to each individual. Understanding what's wrong with the balloon bridges beautifully to recommending treatment and is useful to reference during follow up visits. The model also provides a rationale to patients why their treatment differs from others.

Figure 5.1: The balloon model illustration

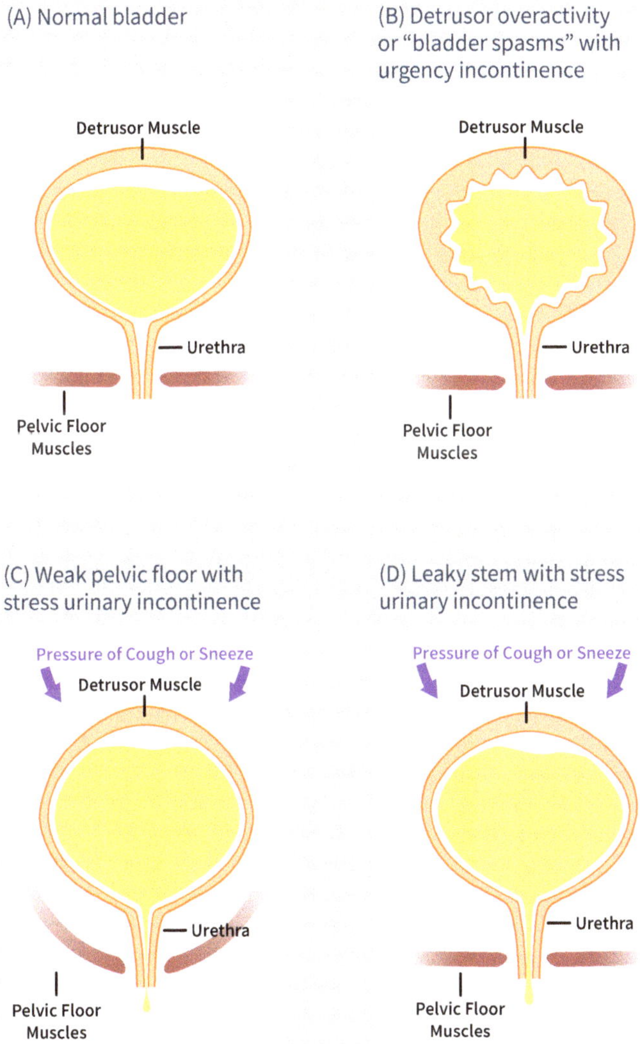

Discussing the balloon model

While using appropriate hand gestures, I explain the balloon model to patients by saying the following:

The bladder works like a balloon. In order to be continent, the balloon fills and the stem is shut. During voiding, the balloon contracts and the stem opens. It's that simple.

Female patients

In women, three things go wrong with the balloon, resulting in urinary incontinence:

- As the balloon fills, it involuntarily contracts or goes into spasm. This results in urgency and urgency incontinence.

- The pelvic floor is a hammock that holds up the balloon. If weakened, when you cough or sneeze, the hammock drops, the balloon drops, the stem opens, and you experience stress incontinence.

- And even if the balloon is well supported by the pelvic floor, if the balloon has a leaky stem, it will also leak with coughing and sneezing.

I then summarize by saying:

So women can have bladder spasms, loss of support, or a leaky stem as the cause of their urinary incontinence. And many have a combination of these problems, resulting in mixed incontinence.

If the patient has an elevated post-void residual, I also include:

A small percentage of women have a fourth reason why they leak. Some women don't empty well, and the bladder spills over like a full glass. Poor emptying of the bladder also aggravates the other three causes just mentioned.

Male patients

In men, 3 things go wrong with the balloon, resulting in loss of urine:

- During filling, the balloon involuntarily contracts or goes into spasm causing urgency and urgency incontinence.

- Following prostate surgery, many men have a leaky stem, and they leak with coughing, sneezing, and with activity.

- Some men don't empty well, and their bladder overflows like a full glass, resulting in incontinence.

It was during my fellowship that I learned the benefits and practical applications of the balloon model. It keeps me focused regardless of the complexity of the problem, and enables me to educate and interact with patients better. Truly a priceless tip from my wonderful friend and mentor, George Webster, MD.

CHAPTER 6

Clinical Evaluation of the Lower Urinary Tract

The clinical evaluation of the lower urinary tract begins with an in-depth history and physical examination. It is the basis of the working diagnosis and directs us to a number of potential investigations and management.

When it comes to the history and physical, we believe that details matter. Certain signs and symptoms, when combined with subsequent evaluation, separate one patient and potentially their treatment pathway from others. Symptom severity, the most bothersome complaint, and what are the patient's treatment goals and expectations are all important aspects to consider.

Especially in the world of electronic medical records (EMR) and an increasing bias towards cut-and-pasted notations, we encourage providers to be careful not to sacrifice the quality of their H&P. Complex voiding dysfunction presented in the medical record only as hourly frequency, recurrent UTI's, and mixed incontinence without other details is of limited value in delivering optimal patient care.

Templates narrow the spectrum of patient variability and complexity, condensing them into a few homogenous groups. They may categorize different individuals as the same nail that, in turn, may be treated with the same hammer. In contrast, the art of managing patients with voiding dysfunction begins with a more representative and individualized patient characterization.

We encourage a focused history and physical that can quickly and efficiently dissect the patient's clinically relevant details. When combined with other diagnostic testing, an effective treatment pathway can be prescribed. In the next two chapters, let's discuss the pertinent aspects of the voiding dysfunction history and physical examination.

Following, we will vet a number of tests that should be liberally used as part of the basic evaluation of patients with voiding dysfunction. These include urinalysis and urine culture, post-void residual urine volume, a bladder diary, and uroflowmetry.

Later on we will dive deeply into the role of more invasive urodynamic testing, endoscopy, and imaging in the LUTS patient.

The Voiding Dysfunction History

An efficient and thorough history provides a representative picture of each unique patient and how their symptoms are affecting their quality of life. It's the first step in the diagnosis to treatment pathway.

Stress urinary incontinence

Patients with stress urinary incontinence (SUI) leak with coughing, sneezing, bending, and lifting. They leak with physical exertion and often limit activity in order to compensate. Is it daily, is it bothersome, and how much do they leak with stress maneuvers are all important questions.

A woman who leaks a few drops playing tennis and who is otherwise continent is different from one who soaks multiple pads daily and leaks during most activities and even walking. "Stress incontinence" as the sole representation in the medical record does not adequately characterize either patient.

Overactive bladder syndrome

Overactive bladder syndrome (OAB) is defined as urinary urgency, usually with urinary frequency and nocturia, with or without urgency urinary incontinence.

The driving symptom of overactive bladder is urinary urgency. *Urgency* is the complaint of a sudden compelling desire to pass urine, which is difficult to defer and can be very disruptive to the patient's quality of life.[13]

Frequency is the complaint by the patient who considers that he/she voids too often. Voiding eight or more times per day was the older ICS definition.

The severity of the overactive bladder is important to ascertain. For example, a patient who voids every 45–60 minutes, and who cannot sit through a two-hour movie because of urgency and frequency, has impressive OAB. The "movie" scenario is a good question to ask patients who provide less clear responses.

For those with severe frequency, it's important to identify the sensation that is driving the behavior in order to differentiate an OAB patient from one with bladder pain syndrome (BPS). Patients voiding frequently because of fullness or urgency should be differentiated from those with BPS, who often urinate in hope to relieve pressure or pain.

Nocturia is waking at night to pass urine. It's the number of voids recorded during a night's sleep, with each void being preceded and followed by sleep. Although voiding once at night is considered abnormal, the literature supports that two or more nighttime voids negatively impacts quality of life. The majority of patients with nocturia have nocturnal polyuria. Other causes of nighttime frequency include high fluid intake, ankle edema, diuretics, heart failure, uncontrolled diabetes, sleep apnea, and sleeping disturbances.

Urgency urinary incontinence is the involuntary loss of urine associated with urgency and an overactive detrusor. It's often triggered approaching the toilet or when going from a sitting to standing position. Other triggers include running water, cold temperatures, key-in-the-door syndrome, and foot-on-the-floor syndrome. Patients who awaken with urgency and leak all the way to the restroom in the middle of the night have OAB and not stress incontinence.

Other presentations of detrusor overactivity

There are a number of other presentations of detrusor overactivity that are clinically relevant but less heralded (Figure 7.1). High volume or flooding incontinence with urine running down the leg, especially if the patient otherwise reports mild or no SUI, is one example. Similarly, giggle incontinence in young women is usually from triggering detrusor overactivity while laughing.

Figure 7.1 Other presentations of detrusor overactivity
Flooding incontinence
Giggle incontinence
Enuresis
Incontinence not associated with awareness
Incontinence during intercourse
Orgasmic related incontinence
Feeling of incomplete emptying
Double voiding pattern
Reduced flow
Post-void dribbling

Enuresis, the involuntary loss of urine while sleeping, is due to an overactive detrusor in most adults. It's a challenging symptom to treat, and grading enuresis as mild, moderate, or severe is beneficial. Bedwetting is made worse by any associated nocturnal diuresis. Some patients with SUI may report enuresis if they cough a lot during sleeping.

Urinary incontinence not associated with awareness is a common complaint. The underlying bladder dysfunction is generally one of three. Severe sphincteric weakness may cause insensate urine loss, but the patient will usually have significant SUI identified by history, physical, and urodynamics. Overflow incontinence is less common in women and identified by measuring the post-void residual. Finally, an overactive detrusor contraction not perceived as urgency is common in the elderly and those with reduced bladder sensation.

Incontinence during intercourse is a distressing symptom, often motivating the patient to seek treatment. Urine loss associated with thrusting is usually due to urethral sphincteric weakness. Spontaneous leakage that is sometimes associated with urgency and high volume, and one that continues in spite of partner withdrawal is likely due to triggered detrusor overactivity. Urine loss during orgasm is also believed to be secondary to an overactive detrusor.

Patients with OAB commonly complain of voiding symptoms. *A feeling of incomplete emptying and a double-voiding pattern* are often associated with a hypersensitive bladder. Some perform positional changes in an attempt to feel empty.

A *reduced flow* is reported by many. Once named small volume frequency syndrome, the urinary flow rate is dependent on bladder volume. A sudden urgency experienced at low volumes prematurely sends the patient to the restroom. The contraction abates prior to voiding, resulting in urinary hesitancy, poor flow, stopping and starting, and straining during attempts to void a small amount. The patient may have a stronger flow first thing in the morning or following prolonged intervals of bladder filling.

The etiology of *post-void dribbling* is poorly understood, and may be due to an after contraction that is sometimes demonstrated during urodynamics in patients with OAB. It may also occur from delay or deficiency in urethral coaptation at the end of urination. Other causes include urethral diverticulum, poor urinary flow, and vaginal voiding.

Mixed stress and urgency incontinence

Mixed stress and urgency incontinence is the complaint of urine loss associated with urgency, and also with exertion, sneezing, coughing, or effort. The stress component is usually easy to identify, while the presentation of detrusor overactivity is more vast and variable. Identifying which component is most severe, or whether both aspects are significant, should be determined. In our experience, the overactive detrusor is often dominant in mixed patients, especially those who are older or have severe symptoms.

Symptom severity

Quantitating the severity of urinary incontinence is part of the evaluation. Identifying the number of pads used daily and whether they are usually damp, moderately wet, or soaked is beneficial. Recognizing its subjectiveness, this simple evaluation is still informative.

A mixed patient soaking eight heavy pads per day primarily related to urgency is different from one using three damp liners in order to control their mixed incontinence occurring mainly with activity. Remember, an H&P noting only "mixed urinary incontinence" and cut and pasted throughout the medical record does not adequately describe either patient.

Quantitating the severity of urinary incontinence is part of the evaluation. Identifying the number of pads used daily and whether they are usually damp, moderately wet, or soaked is beneficial. Recognizing its subjectiveness, this simple evaluation is still informative.

Voiding symptoms

Voiding symptoms are common, especially in males with lower urinary tract symptoms attributed to benign prostatic hyperplasia (BPH).

Slow stream is reported when the patient's perceived urine flow is reduced, usually compared to previous performance or in comparison to others.

Asking if a patient's flow is good, poor, or reasonable helps identify the symptom recognizing that in many individuals the flow varies. Patients often respond, "sometimes good, sometimes poor," which is understandable given the flow variation that occurs during different times of the day or night. An isolated strong flow that only occurs with urgency may be being generated by an overactive detrusor contraction.

Urinary hesitancy is the term used when an individual describes difficulty in initiating micturition, resulting in a delay in the onset of voiding after the individual is ready to pass urine. Standing and even sitting for several moments before voiding is common in obstructed patients and in those having difficulty relaxing their external urethral sphincter and pelvic floor in order to urinate.

Intermittency is the term used when the individual describes a urine flow which stops and starts during micturition. It is important to determine whether the pattern is associated with straining, as it may signify poor bladder contractility or severe bladder outlet obstruction. Intermittency is also reported in those with external sphincter dyssynergia.

Spraying of urination may identify the presence of a urethral stricture, especially one close to the urethral meatus. Prior urethral instrumentation, catheterization, sexually transmitted diseases, and surgery are all risk factors for urethral stricture and should be noted.

Having discussed the most common lower urinary tract symptoms, other aspects of the voiding dysfunction history deserve attention. A more detailed account of each may be revisited in the Diagnosis to Treatment Pathway Modules.

Recurrent urinary tract infections

The diagnosis of recurrent urinary tract infections (UTI's) is important to establish, especially in women with OAB or pelvic pain complaints. Although there is an agreed upon definition of recurrent UTI's, there has been a notorious misuse of the term by patients and providers. Consequently, a devil's advocate approach is advised before accepting the diagnosis.

It's important to ask patients to describe their typical UTI symptoms. In many cases the symptoms are vague and nonspecific. Be suspect of those who report that they are "always infected." Whether or not the patient says that their symptoms temporarily respond to antibiotics is a good clue. Others may reference previous positive cultures, or that their provider called them back to switch their antibiotics. Being admitted for urosepsis or given parenteral antibiotics for a UTI and sent home by the Emergency Department is not confirmatory. Often lab follow-up of these events demonstrates a negative or absent urine culture.

In addition to improving quality of life with effective management, the elimination of UTI's can benefit the patient's chronic voiding symptoms. Overactive bladder and pelvic pain commonly down-regulate and improve once UTI's have been prevented with long-term suppressive antibiotics. Even vague lower abdominal, back, and vaginal complaints may normalize with down-regulation.

A sound principle to follow is that you must control multiple recurrent UTI's before you can successfully control urinary incontinence. Urinary symptoms temporarily worsen with each infection but may continue even after successful treatment. Ongoing or new OAB medications may be much more effective once the UTI's are prevented.

Pelvic organ prolapse

We are familiar with the symptoms associated with pelvic organ prolapse (POP), including a vaginal bulge or uncomfortable pressure that is worse while standing or sitting. The patient often reports touching or seeing something near or beyond the vaginal introitus. Other descriptions include spontaneous or digital reduction of the prolapse and splinting maneuvers to assist voiding or defecation.

Symptoms commonly reported but often not related to POP include suprapubic pressure, vague abdominal complaints, and back pain. Rectoceles do not cause diarrhea, constipation, and other functional bowel symptoms. Pain with intercourse is likely due to vaginal atrophy or other factors, and is usually not due to POP. Blocked intercourse or mild discomfort during penetration is likely related.

Identifying what symptoms are most bothersome and establishing treatment goals and expectations is important prior to recommending diagnostic testing and therapy. Many women with prolapse are primarily troubled by unrelated bladder symptoms, while others are just seeking reassurance.

It's noteworthy how some women feel and are bothered by objectively mild prolapse, while others, often elderly or obese, are asymptomatic in spite of advanced stage POP. Bothersome symptoms and not the degree of prolapse should dictate management.

Vaginal atrophy and associated discomfort when successfully treated by local hormone replacement therapy can be effective in managing milder prolapse symptoms. Vaginal pressure and the sensation that something is falling out can vanish once the vaginal epithelium is re-estrogenized. Dyspareunia similarly can improve with estrogen and physical therapy and the prolapse managed conservatively.

Bladder pain syndrome

The ICS defines interstitial cystitis/bladder pain syndrome (IC/BPS) as "the complaint of suprapubic pain related to bladder filling, accompanied by other symptoms such as increased daytime and nighttime frequency, in the absence of proven urinary infection or other obvious pathology."

Typically, these patients void frequently in an attempt to relieve pelvic pressure or pain and not due to urgency and fear of incontinence. Symptoms are commonly relieved by voiding, but in some cases the pain worsens or remains unchanged.

Symptom flares unresponsive to antibiotics, waxing and waning or cyclical complaints, and dyspareunia may suggest IC/BPS. The diagnosis should be considered in those voiding several times per hour, especially when associated with the sensation of incomplete emptying, even in the absence of pain. Many with IC/BPS have associated anxiety, bowel complaints, fibromyalgia, headaches, or other pain syndromes.

Those with IC/BPS may report urethral discomfort and dysuria and be diagnosed as having urethritis. Perhaps just a terminology issue, inflammation in the bladder can refer pain to many locations including the urethra, abdomen, lower back, and vagina. Isolated vaginal burning in the absence of other pathology can sometimes be the presenting symptom.

Neurogenic lower urinary tract dysfunction

Patients with neurologic disorders are at risk of having lower urinary tract dysfunction, and are commonly seen in a tertiary referral practice. The nature of the dysfunction generally depends on the neurologic disease, as well as the presence of any underlying bladder condition.

Patients who present with urinary symptoms out of the ordinary should be suspect of having a non-diagnosed neurologic disorder. A thirty-eight-year-old man who keeps a urinal in his truck to manage his urinary frequency or a teenage woman with enuresis and flooding urgency incontinence is not normal. The acute onset of incontinence or other voiding complaints in the absence of other causes should also alert one to the possibility of a neurologic etiology.

Patients who present with urinary symptoms out of the ordinary should be suspected of having a non-diagnosed neurologic disorder.

When suspect, the presence of other neurologic symptoms should be looked for. Vaginal or perineal numbness, diminished sensation during intercourse, voiding or defecation, the presence of fecal incontinence, symptoms suggesting sciatica, transient loss of vision, vague neurologic extremity complaints, and many others may be suggestive.

Urinary incontinence not associated with awareness can occur in those with neurologically impaired bladder sensation. Those with reduced sensation may report voiding on a timed schedule and not based upon bladder fullness. Others don't feel the need to urinate first thing in the morning despite them having a full bladder.

In patients performing clean intermittent catheterization (CIC) it's important to determine the frequency of CIC and its measured or estimated volume. Leaking between catheterization from detrusor overactivity may be volume dependent and secondary to high fluid intake or a nocturnal diuresis, which is common in wheelchair patients with dependent lower leg edema.

An understanding of the neurologic disease helps providers manage patients with neurogenic lower urinary tract dysfunction. The condition's natural history and how it may affect bladder and overall functional status now and in the future is paramount, especially when considering invasive and irreversible therapies. Some patients lose hand function or experience deteriorating mental status as their disease progresses.

Bowel dysfunction

The majority of urologists and many gynecologists have limited expertise in managing bowel dysfunction. Having said that, identification of the presence of fecal urgency, frequency, and incontinence are basic to understanding pelvic floor function.

The presence of bowel dysfunction should be considered when recommending a diagnosis to treatment pathway. The side effects of antimuscarinics could affect baseline function and sacral neuromodulation is approved for fecal incontinence. The neurologic cross talk between bowel and bladder is widely accepted and improving bowel function can secondarily help urinary symptoms, especially in children and the elderly. Constipation and other anal disorders can precipitate urinary retention.

Timing of symptoms

The timing and onset of lower urinary tract symptoms is often relevant. For example, a 53-year-old male with LUTS dating back two decades is not suffering from BPH. A woman with a life-long history of overactive bladder will likely have persistent OAB following a sling that was performed for a more recent development of mixed incontinence. A new onset of incontinence in a male who was initially dry for years after his prostatectomy is more likely due to detrusor overactivity and not SUI.

The acute onset of symptoms should encourage one to look for a precipitating cause, such as a urinary tract infection, constipation, a new medication or medical event, etc. Remember that acute changes in bladder function can be secondary to a number of intravesical causes including carcinoma.

The temporal relationship of symptoms relative to a potential precipitant has diagnostic implications and may influence treatment recommendations. De novo symptoms following a bladder neck suspension, spinal cord surgery, a stroke, or similar event are likely related. A careful history of bladder function before and after the incident is necessary. We caution against blaming more distant events recognizing that many patients are biased to do so when in fact they are not related.

General urologic history

A number of general urologic questions is part of the voiding dysfunction evaluation. Previous surgery of the lower urinary tract, a history of malignancy, radiation therapy, hysterectomy, hematuria, fluid intake, and general health survey, to name a few.

Regarding past surgical history, there are several important issues to realize. A previous open retropubic bladder suspension may predispose to the presence of retropubic scarring, making future dissection more challenging. The bladder neck and proximal urethra were often overcorrected by these procedures, causing worsening of the lower urinary tract symptoms. The presence of pelvic or abdominal mesh should be determined, since it may complicate therapy is some patients.

The Voiding Dysfunction Physical Examination

Findings during the physical examination are often clinically relevant and allow us to separate one patient from another. Just as with history-taking, we caution against using computerized templates that condense many patients into a standardized physical exam at the expense of important and often nuanced findings.

Female examination

Stress incontinence

When assessing women with SUI, there are several findings during the pelvic examination that can influence treatment decision making, such as degree of urethral hypermobility, cough stress test, amount of urine loss, and the presence of associated prolapse.

The degree of rotational descent of the urethra is readily visualized on exam without the additional aid of a Q-tip. A fixed urethra, or one with minimal descensus, is different from a hypermobile one, and its presence may influence treatment options.

A positive cough stress test confirms the diagnosis of SUI. Urinary loss that continues for several moments after the cough or Valsalva likely represents a cough-induced overactive detrusor contraction. Spontaneous leakage with insertion or downward depression of a speculum may similarly be from a triggered bladder spasm event. Although rare, in some cases, too much downward traction may distort an already compromised sphincter resulting in stress incontinence.

The amount of urine loss during coughing and Valsalva should be noted, as should the strength or effort of the cough/Valsalva. Leaking a few drops with a hard cough is less severe than high volume leakage generated by a modest Valsalva. Bladder fullness could affect this subjective assessment, and the evaluation can be repeated with a full bladder if cystoscopy is performed at a later date.

An asymptomatic grade II cystocele that descends beyond a less mobile urethra could result in a postoperative obstructing "hinge" effect following a sling for SUI. The altered anatomy may cause or worsen flow symptoms postoperatively. Over time, the repetitive hinging of the prolapse over the mesh could predispose to sling erosion at the level of the bladder neck.

Inspection of the vagina for the presence of other conditions is important when evaluating patients with SUI. Vaginal epithelial folds, elevations, or possible cysts underneath the urethra may represent an asymptomatic urethral diverticulum. Magnetic resonance imaging can confirm the diagnosis and should be performed prior to bladder neck surgery. Video-urodynamics may identify a diverticulum but the false negative rate with fluoroscopy is significant. Vaginal atrophy and epithelial thinning could compromise healing and increase the rate of mesh extrusion. Local estrogen replacement therapy is often helpful prior to surgery.

Mesh extrusion should be looked for in SUI patients who have had previous vaginal mesh. The presence of an over-corrected and elevated urethro-vesical angle and a past history of a retropubic bladder neck suspension may suggest the presence of obstruction.

Body habitus should also be observed in surgical patients. Transvaginal retropubic slings can be safely performed in most obese patients but may be challenging in those with a significant pannus. A trans-obturator or single-incision approach may be more appropriate, but the long-term effectiveness of the latter in this population has not been proven.

Inspection of the vulva and perineum is relevant. The presence of urinary dermatitis suggests long-term high-volume incontinence or inadequate pad usage and poor hygiene. Lichen sclerosis is often bothersome and appropriate management for this is recommended. Evidence of skin changes secondary to pelvic radiation should serve as a reminder not to use mesh in this population.

Pelvic organ prolapse

The examination of pelvic organ prolapse is a learned skill. Excellent lighting and positioning the patient at the end of the table is very helpful. Sometimes it's necessary to have patients stand with one leg mildly separated and elevated on a short stool and bear down in order to identify their prolapse. A patient's ability to cough or to perform a Valsalva varies, and it's best to use which ever one is most effective. Coaching the patient to keep pushing, while simultaneously measuring the degree of apical descensus with one's index finger or measurement device, is a good technique. Direct visualization of the apex during Valsalva while slightly pulling back on the speculum avoids false negative, and is another technique to evaluate for apical descensus.

The lower aspect of the double-bill speculum is used to evaluate prolapse but an intact speculum is often necessary to observe the cervix.

The immediate availability of varying size speculums is recommended. Many elderly women have a narrow vaginal introitus and require a smaller size in order to be examined. Wider and longer speculums can effectively reduce prolapse in woman with very lax and voluminous vaginas.

Identification of the presence of an anterior and posterior defect and vault prolapse is paramount. The diagnosis of an enterocele may be difficult but should be suspected in those with significant posterior apical weakness. The absence of vaginal rugae may help differentiate a smooth enterocele or "double-bubble" from the transverse ridges commonly associated with a rectocele.

Numerous grading systems exist in order to describe the presence and severity of pelvic organ prolapse. The ICS, AUGS, and others endorse and recommend the POP-Q.[14] As an objective measure, it has been successfully used in clinical practice and research.

The likelihood of needing a vault suspension during an anterior or posterior repair should be determined prior to surgery. Providers should be aware that pelvic exam findings may be different under anesthesia when the patient is relaxed. Mild prolapse while awake can be rather significant when examined under anesthesia. Consequently, thorough patient counseling regarding the potential need for additional prolapse repair is warranted.

Vaginal access and length is also important to consider. A narrow introitus and pubic arch in combination with a long vagina and apical defect can be challenging to address vaginally. A prolapsed short vagina can be further compromised when repaired vaginally and may be best treated transabdominally, especially in those who are sexually active. A long voluminous vagina with multiple site defects, sometimes associated with pelvic side wall and introital laxity, may be better managed with a sacral colpopexy. The fixation points associated with a sacrospinous vault suspension may not be deep enough to effectively manage the apex in these patients.

Reducing the prolapse and assessing for SUI is critical. Gently turning the speculum sideways to free the bladder neck while simultaneously reducing the prolapse is a good technique (Figure 8-1). A non-obstructing vaginal pack or ring forceps may also be utilized.

The evaluation of prolapse may help predict the likelihood of successful pessary fitting. In addition, vaginal atrophy should be identified and treated when clinically appropriate. The presence of vaginal ulcers associated with prolapse should be treated prior to surgery.

Figure 8.1:

Reducing the prolapse and assessing for SUI.

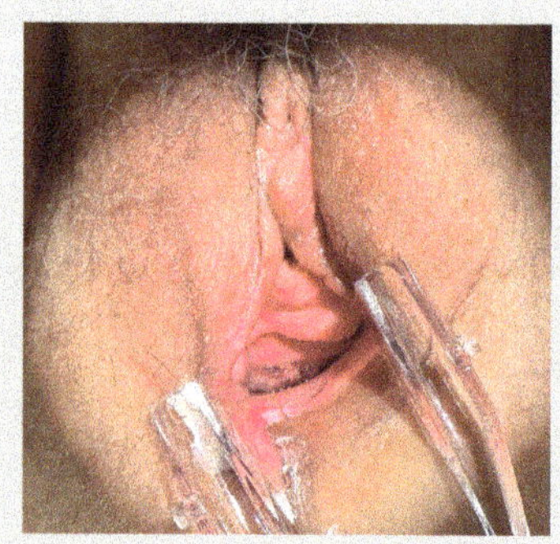

Pelvic pain symptoms

Patients with pelvic pain may demonstrate a number of findings during physical examination. The presence of vaginal atrophy, vaginitis, a urethral diverticulum, or Skene's gland cyst can be readily observed. Patients with IC/BPS often have tight and tender levator pelvic floor muscles and are sensitive to gentle palpation of the introitus and bladder. Other trigger points in these hyper-esthetic patients include the abdomen, back, and suprapubic area. Similarly, IC/BPS patients may be uncomfortable with urethral instrumentation or with bladder filling during cystoscopy.

Urinary flow symptoms

Many women with voiding dysfunction have urinary flow symptoms. They report urinary hesitancy, stopping and starting, and using positional changes to assist in urination. Others lean back, lift up on their lower abdomen, or perform a Credé maneuver to void. In many cases the symptoms are due to pelvic floor dyssynergia which may be suggested by having tight or tender levator muscles on physical examination. The presence of a large cystocele, meatal stenosis, a diverticulum or Skene's gland cyst, and an over-corrected bladder neck should also be looked for.

Digital rectal examination (DRE)

Although female DRE is rarely performed by most urologists, it has relevant purpose for evaluation of pelvic floor, bowel, and sexual function. It may help identify the severity of a rectocele, the presence of perineal laxity, and the degree of constipation. Anal sphincteric function can be assessed in those with fecal incontinence and rectal prolapse can be diagnosed.

Male examination

The examination in men with urinary incontinence is important especially when considering surgery. Men with SUI following a prostatectomy commonly demonstrate a positive cough test in the standing position. A negative test likely represents milder incontinence or a relatively empty bladder during the exam. High urine loss that continues to leak long after the cough subsides may be due to significant urethral incompetence or cough-induced detrusor overactivity.

When considering an artificial urinary sphincter, the presence of an inguinal hernia should be looked for and the reservoir placed on the contralateral side if one exists. Changing sides to avoid abdominal mesh is similarly recommended. A high riding scrotum with a large protuberant abdomen may make cycling an artificial sphincter challenging to the patient. Hand pincer function should be assessed in those with significant arthritis or neurologic disease. Scrotal skin conditions such as urinary dermatitis need to be treated prior to placement of a sphincter or male sling.

Neurogenic bladder examination

In patients suspected of having a neurogenic bladder, the presence of vaginal, scrotal, and perineal numbness should be evaluated. Loss of passive and voluntary anal sphincter control could exist. Depending on the underlying neurologic disorder, a number of sensory and motor findings in the extremities may be demonstrated. In younger patients, examination of the lower back for stigmata suggesting spinal bifida occulta and palpation for sacral agenesis is recommended.

Functional assessment

A cursory assessment of the patient's functional physical and mental status is part of the initial evaluation. For example, the presence of a walker, a cane or wheelchair, or a home-oxygen tank are noteworthy and may influence evaluation and treatment recommendations.

Don't be embarrassed to approach the diagnosis of memory loss and one's ability to self-toilet with the patient or family member. A quick look at the referring records may reveal the diagnosis of dementia. The presence of significant medical comorbidities should also be taken into consideration.

Patient behavior

Untoward patient behavior should be documented in the medical record. We now live in a world in which patient anxiety, anger, finger-pointing, and unrealistic expectations are reality, and managing some of these patients can be challenging.

Getting to know patients prior to recommending surgery is beneficial. A good rule is try not to operate on the first date and don't ignore red flags, especially when they recur. Be cautious of patients who "just want it fixed" or who are overly reluctant to first try conservative approaches. Other warning signs include patients who appear acutely distraught about their condition even though they have had it for years. Be careful operating on those who don't appear to be listening well or understanding your recommendations. Words matter and inappropriate comments to you, your nurses, or front-desk staff should be noted as they are potential red flags.

Many of these patients can be very upset when surgery does not reach their treatment goal or if they experience a complication. History has taught us that litigation associated with pelvic floor surgery must be taken seriously by all. Do not be afraid to back away from a surgical candidate who has demonstrated red flags. Words calmly spoken by my mentor to the sometimes difficult patient, "I'm sorry, I don't think I will be able to reach your treatment goal," with or without a referral to another physician, is recommended wisdom.

Untoward patient behavior should be documented in the medical record. We now live in a world in which patient anxiety, anger, finger-pointing, and unrealistic expectations are reality, and managing some of these patients can be challenging.

Diagnostic Stethoscopes

In addition to an in-depth history and physical examination, there are a number of basic tests that should be liberally used as part of the initial evaluation of patients with voiding dysfunction. We sometimes refer to these tests as our diagnostic stethoscopes. These stethoscopes include urinalysis and urine culture, post-void residual urine volume, a bladder diary, and uroflowmetry (Figure 9.1).

Figure 9.1 Diagnostic stethoscopes
Urinalysis and culture
Post-void residual urine volume
Bladder diary
Uroflowmetry

Urinalysis and urine culture

Most providers routinely obtain a urinalysis as part of the basic evaluation in patients with voiding dysfunction. The presence of microscopic hematuria, glucosuria, or suggestion of infection are markers for underlying disease. Unfortunately urine cultures have been underused and undervalued. We believe that the liberal use of urine cultures significantly impacts the treatment of many patients.

Patients with any voiding dysfunction should have consideration of a UTI as either a primary source or ancillary contributor. Unexplained worsening urinary frequency and incontinence, severe incontinence in the elderly, several months of vague storage or voiding complaints, acute or chronic pelvic pain and pressure are all examples of patients who may have a UTI in the absence of "cystitis" symptoms. Even in the presence of having a normal or mildly abnormal urinalysis, many of them will have a causal positive culture and respond favorably when treated.

Women with overactive bladder may have positive cultures but otherwise be asymptomatic. They are historically diagnosed as having asymptomatic bacteriuria when in fact their "low grade infection" is worsening or causing the symptoms. The up-regulation of voiding dysfunction and pelvic pain occurs secondary to bacteriuria. The inflammatory response by the urothelium to inciting local bacteria can chronically up-regulate sensory urgency or pain pathways. For instance, a post-UTI bladder hypersensitivity is a diagnosis in which a once normal bladder was upregulated by a UTI and then it remains irritated and inflamed despite effective treatment of the infection.

For instance, a post-UTI bladder hypersensitivity is a diagnosis in which a once normal bladder was upregulated by a UTI and then it remains irritated and inflamed despite effective treatment of the infection.

Positive urine cultures in voiding dysfunction patients should be considered as part of the problem. Having been diagnosed with recurrent UTI's or chronic occult cystitis, many of these patients, when successfully treated and then suppressed by prophylactic antibiotics or other therapies, eventually down-regulate. Treating their "asymptomatic bacteriuria" can surprisingly have impressive long-lasting results. The length of antibiotic suppression is unknown, but a trial of six to twelve months is reasonable. If the symptom complex returns upon cessation of prophylaxis, the same treatment algorithm can be applied again but for longer-term. It's noteworthy how often the lower urinary tract dysfunction diagnosis to treatment pathway is changed when one is cognizant of the role of bacteriuria in this population.

A few additional tips regarding urine cultures deserve mentioning. It is beneficial to obtain a urine culture in patients with a Foley catheter who are undergoing a trial of voiding. Recognizing that the urine is likely colonized and typically left untreated, it's nice to have a culture available if the patient calls a few days later with symptoms suggestive of a UTI. Many who pass their voiding trial still have elevated residuals, which may make the bacteriuria problematic. We treat positive cultures in this population.

It's recommended to obtain a culture 7–10 days prior to implantation of an artificial sphincter or male sling, and to treat if postive. Exposing an implant or mesh to bacteriuria could have a devastating impact even when preoperative intravenous antibiotics are given. Relying on symptoms and a normal preoperative urinalysis may miss a rare bacteriuria and is not recommended as the sole criteria.

We commonly diagnose patients with prostatitis, urethritis, a Skene's gland cyst, an infected urethral diverticulum, and similar. Even though the urine culture is often negative they should be ordered initially and during recurrent symptomatic flares. When positive, the urine culture can better direct effective management.

Distinguishing patients with recurrent UTI's from those suffering from bladder pain syndrome can be difficult based on past history. Getting urine cultures during symptom flares on patients placed on daily antibiotic prophylaxis will help provide the diagnosis. A happy asymptomatic patient after many months of suppressive therapy highly suggests a previous diagnosis of UTI's. Recurrent flares with negative cultures in the same patient on prophylaxis likely indicates interstitial cystitis.

In a patient who presents with LUTS and suspected colonization, a trial of antibiotics is recommended. It's important to identify which symptom you are treating and whether or not it improves following therapy. Close follow up is important to measure the response. Many women are colonized with streptococcus which is often non-virulent and does not need treatment. However, if acute UTI symptoms arise or are noted in patients with long-term chronic voiding complaints, it is recommended to treat and assess treatment outcome. Occasionally, this management strategy will resolve symptoms.

Post-void residual

Determination of the post-void residual (PVR) urine volume by bladder scanner, ultrasound, and, less often, with a catheter is beneficial in assessing patients with voiding dysfunction (Figure 9.2).

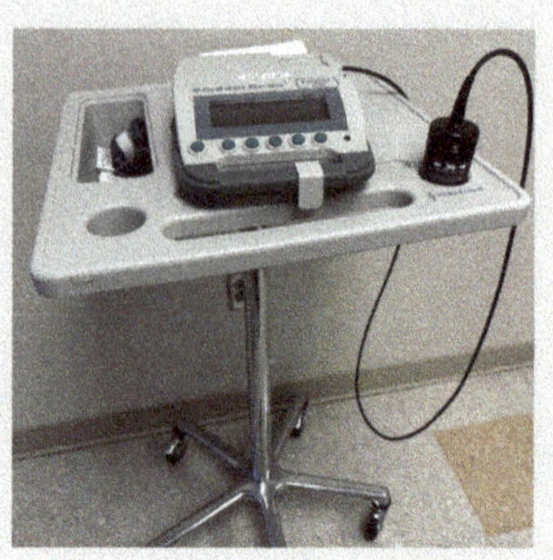

Figure 9.2 Bladder Scanner
The bladder scanner measures the post-void residual (PVR). The PVR is determined prior to seeing the patient.

The Adult Urodynamics AUA/SUFU Guidelines recommend:

Guidelines

A PVR in women with SUI considering invasive therapy, those patients suspect of having a neurogenic bladder, and in male LUTS patients as a safety measure to rule out significant retention initially and in follow-up.

Surprisingly, no other guideline statements regarding PVR are published.

In contrast, we recommend a PVR in the majority of patients with voiding dysfunction. All men and women with incontinence regardless of type, day or nighttime frequency, flow symptoms, pelvic pressure or pain, and recurrent UTI's should be assessed. The presence of an elevated residual in these patients has diagnostic and therapeutic relevance.

The definition of an elevated PVR has not been clearly established but most accept a value > 100 mL as being abnormal, and one that is greater than 50 mL might prompt the suspicion of voiding dysfunction.

Comparing the residual volume to the voided volume helps put the PVR into clinical perspective. For example, a residual of 140 mL in a patient who voids 800 mL may have less consequence than in an OAB patient who voids small amounts and who has a low functional bladder capacity.

We agree with the guidelines that elevated PVR's should be repeated to rule out false positives. Many patients are asked to void prematurely or void less efficiently in public. Those with high residuals should be routinely asked if their void was representative of normal. Having them try to double void without straining followed by rescanning is useful.

The Adult Urodynamics AUA/SUFU Guidelines recommend a PVR in women with SUI considering invasive therapy, those patients suspect of having a neurogenic bladder, and in male LUTS patients as a safety measure to rule out significant retention initially and in follow-up.

A falsely elevated residual is commonly seen during the unnatural setting of urodynamics. The physiologic PVR, measured during the initial office visit, is often the best reading. If needed, patients should return for a follow-up with a comfortably full bladder to ascertain an accurate assessment.

Figure 9.3 Elevated PVR on scanner

Elevated PVR in a woman with lower urinary tract symptoms. Recommended follow-up questions include:
1. Was the void representative of your normal?
2. Do you feel like you have emptied your bladder?
3. Are you able to void a second time, and if yes, I will rescan you?

Answers are documented in the medical record.

```
BladderScan(tm)
  01/27/22    09:37

 226ml
```

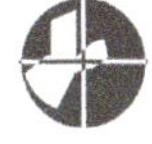

```
FEMALE
Patient name:

- - - - - - - - - - - - - - - - - -

Patient ID:

- - - - - - - - - - - - - - - - - -

Procedure code:

- - - - - - - - - - - - - - - - - -

Signature:

- - - - - - - - - - - - - - - - - -
```

Our staff obtains the urinalysis and PVR prior to the provider interviewing the patient. Knowing the residual may influence the focus of the history and physical in real time. An elevated PVR may represent obstruction, and is sometimes a surrogate marker for poor bladder contractility. This is especially the case when the high residual is not associated with a sensation of bladder fullness. Depending on the patient's presentation, an elevated PVR is an indication for pressure-flow urodynamics.

The presence of silent hydronephrosis should be considered in those with high residuals. Although there is no predictive cut-off, it is reasonable to perform a screening renal ultrasound in those with residuals > 200–300 mL.

Patients with elevated residuals should be followed to detect early silent bladder decompensation and/or hydronephrosis over time. Fortunately, clean intermittent catheterization is rarely indicated. It is generally accepted that a markedly elevated PVR is a risk factor for UTI's, upper tract deterioration, and stone disease. These patients deserve upper tract evaluation and close long-term surveillance.

Bladder diary

Bladder diaries are a simple, noninvasive tool used in the evaluation of patients with voiding dysfunction, especially those with storage symptoms and urinary incontinence. They provide an excellent natural urodynamic record of bladder function.

Bladder diaries record the time and volume of each micturition, providing an objective assessment of the number of daytime and nighttime voids, as well as 24-hour frequency. The maximum voided volume during a single micturition is a reasonable indicator of the patient's awake functional bladder capacity.

Self-monitoring for 3–7 days is generally recommended in OAB studies, but patient compliance and inconvenience must be considered in clinical practice. We recommend recording for 24–48 hours. A diary and measuring apparatus are provided to each patient, along with simple instructions. If workdays are unrealistic for recording, we encourage weekend monitoring.

The number of urinary incontinence episodes and whether they are associated with a stress maneuver or urgency are noted. More elaborate diaries demonstrate the presence and severity of urinary urgency.

Noting the time and amount of fluid intake provides important diagnostic information demonstrating how lifestyle can influence voiding patterns. Polyuria, generally accepted as a 24-hour urine volume of greater than 40 mL/Kg, is often secondary to high fluid intake.

Diagnostic patterns

From a diagnostic standpoint, there are a number of voiding patterns demonstrated on diaries that are clinically useful.

Patients with overactive bladder, once coined small volume frequency syndrome, typically void frequent small amounts and commonly demonstrate significant variation in voided volumes. It's impressive how an overactive detrusor can signal to a patient that their bladder is full at such low volumes. Patient realization of this is an important beginning of an effective bladder retraining program (Figure 9.4).

Figure 9.4 Bladder diary – overactive bladder

Urinary frequency and urgency incontinence in a male patient with overactive bladder. His voided volumes are low and vary.

Date	Time am/pm	Fluid Intake ml/oz	Volume Voided ml/oz	Leaks (check space)
	8:15 am		210	
	9:20 am		140	
	10:45 am			✓ Urgency
	11:10 am		70	
	12:50 pm		110	
	2:00 pm		225	
	2:45 pm			✓ Urgency
	3:40 pm		130	
	5:15 pm		40	
	6:00 pm		70	
	7:15 pm		215	
	10:30 pm		160	
	2:00 am		80	
	7:00 am		165	

Patients with severe frequency and a markedly reduced functional capacity should be suspected of having a hypersensitive detrusor. Interstitial cystitis/bladder pain syndrome (IC/BPS) or reduced bladder capacity secondary to fibrosis may be present. Typically, these patients tend to have less variability in their volume voided and many urinate more than once per hour. A low bladder capacity measured under anesthesia or the presence of glomerulations after hydrodistension can confirm the diagnosis.

Bladder diaries are the mainstay in diagnosing nocturia secondary to a nocturnal diuresis. The ICS defines nocturnal polyuria as a nocturnal urine output > 33% of the daily total in patients older than 65 years and >20% in younger patients. The literature confirms that nocturnal polyuria is present in the majority of adults voiding two or more times nightly. Similarly, patients with congestive heart failure, dependent edema, uncontrolled diabetes, and sleep apnea commonly have high nocturnal urine production (Figure 9.5).

Many patients presenting with 24-hour storage symptoms have both an overactive bladder and nocturnal diuresis confirmed on their bladder

Figure 9.5 Bladder diary – nocturnal diuresis

Nighttime frequency in a 70-year-old women with nocturnal polyuria. Her nocturnal urine output is > 33% of the daily total.

Date	Time am/pm	Fluid Intake ml/oz	Volume Voided ml/oz	Leaks (check space)
	8:00 am		320	
	9:10 am		280	
	11:40 am		160	
	3:10 pm		290	
	6:40 pm		390	
	8:55 pm		160	
	1:15 am		420	
	3:00 am		375	
	4:45 am		290	
	7:10 am		440	

diary. Their nocturnal polyuria in combination with a small functional bladder capacity clearly explains their significant nighttime symptoms.

As noted, increased frequency of normal voided volumes is typically seen in polyuria patients secondary to high fluid intake. The same pattern is present in those with uncontrolled diabetes mellitus or diabetes insipidus.

Therapeutic value

In addition to aiding in diagnosis, voiding diaries play a role in the treatment of patients with voiding dysfunction. The curtailment of high fluid intake and bladder irritants revealed by self-monitoring can be very beneficial. Diaries provide an objective recording of voiding intervals, and are an excellent cheerleader encouraging interval prolongation during bladder retraining. As a star chart is to a child with enuresis, tracking positive progress with a voiding diary is a helpful addition to behavioral and medical therapy.

Other uses

Some patients with voiding dysfunction are poor historians, and a bladder diary may prove useful as an objective representation of their presenting problem. It also gives urodynamic staff important pretest information regarding anticipated cystometric filling volumes, as well as a possible working diagnosis.

Uroflowmetry

When it comes to patients with voiding symptoms, uroflowmetry is a simple noninvasive test. It electronically measures the rate of flow of voided urine, and is performed using a simple flowmeter.

Uroflowmetry is an excellent screening tool for bladder outlet obstruction (BOO), especially when it's combined with the post-void residual. A reduced flow is also present in those with poor bladder contractility and may be an indication for more extensive urodynamic testing.

Patients are instructed to void normally, either sitting or standing, with a comfortably full bladder and in privacy to reduce the inhibitory effects of the testing environment. Once completed, the patient is asked if the void was representative of his or her usual. Voided volumes of less than 150 mL can lead to erroneous results and should be repeated.

Younger men under 40 years generally have a maximum flow rate (Qmax) of greater than 25mL/s. Flow rates decrease with age and unobstructed men older than 60 years with a normally functioning detrusor usually have flow rates greater that 15 mL/s. Data suggests that approximately 90% of men with LUTS and a Qmax of less than 10 mL/s are obstructed on pressure-flow studies. Normal flow rates in women are less well defined, but are generally 5 to 10 mL/s greater than men for a given bladder volume.

Diagnostic flow patterns

The flow rate and uroflow pattern may give important diagnostic clues to the patient's underlying voiding dysfunction problem (Figure 9.6). A normally functioning and unobstructed detrusor typically generates a smooth bell-shaped uroflow curve with a rapid rise to a high amplitude peak (Qmax). Less important, the time to Qmax should not exceed one-third of the flow time. An exaggeration of the normal curve with a high Qmax is sometimes seen in women with SUI and with low outflow resistance and is commonly referred to as a super voider.

A prolonged depressed flow pattern is frequently seen in BOO and, less commonly, in those with underactive detrusors. The time to reach a low maximum amplitude is prolonged and associated with an extended flow time. The flow curve is usually asymmetric and has a lengthy declining terminal end.

An interrupted spiking pattern secondary to abdominal straining is typically seen in patients with poor bladder contractility and less so in those obstructed. Intermittent external sphincter or pelvic floor dyssynergia may result in a similar finding.

A low Qmax which plateaus for a prolonged time in a "box-like" fashion may suggest the diagnosis of a urethral stricture. In the presence of a normal detrusor, most strictures remain asymptomatic until the urethral caliber approaches 11 French.

Figure 9.6: Four Diagnostic Flow Patterns

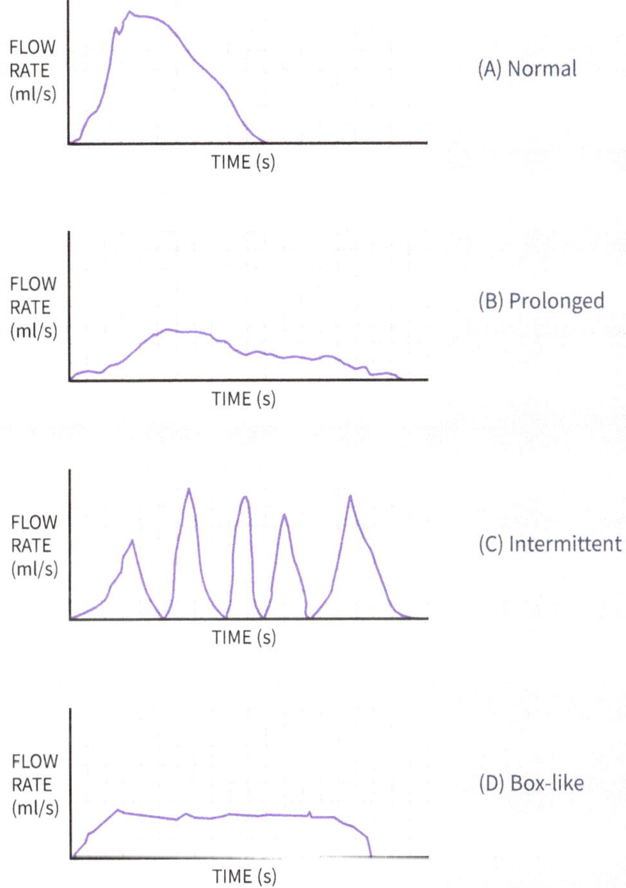

Spiking artifacts due to straining or variations in direction of the urinary stream are commonly noted during uroflowmetry (Figure 9.7). Subsequently, the maximum flow rate electronically recorded may be misleading. Examining the pattern and manually "smoothing" the curve is necessary in order to accurately determine the Qmax in these situations.

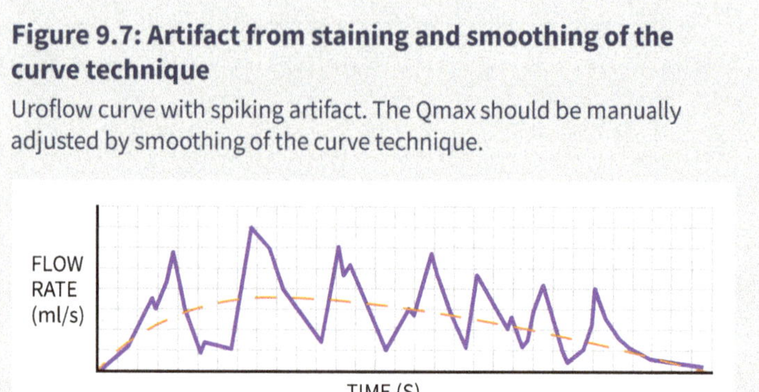

Figure 9.7: Artifact from staining and smoothing of the curve technique

Uroflow curve with spiking artifact. The Qmax should be manually adjusted by smoothing of the curve technique.

Clinical application

There are a number of circumstances when the uroflow findings may bring pause when evaluating patients with voiding dysfunction, such as when it provides a subtle signal that the proposed therapy may be less effective or associated with a complication.

Be careful performing a transurethral resection of the prostate or corresponding office-based procedure in a LUTS patient who has a normal Qmax and flow pattern. Yes, high voiding pressure and normal flow patients do exist, but we recommend pressure-flow urodynamics to confirm the diagnosis. Unobstructed patients generally do less favorably with invasive prostate-directed therapy.

Similarly, male LUTS patients demonstrating a straining spiking uroflow pattern may have a poorly contractile bladder only identified by urodynamics. A large hyposensitive bladder associated with myogenic failure, especially combined with a high residual, is more likely to fail prostate surgery.

Men with flow symptoms and a "box-like" pattern may have a urethral stricture and should undergo cystoscopy. If present, a retrograde urethrogram will help demonstrate stricture caliber and length.

Women with stress incontinence undergoing a bladder neck suspension are at risk of postoperative urinary retention. Unproven, it is reassuring when the patient has a reasonably normal Qmax and flow pattern prior to surgery. Women with flow symptoms and a straining or depressed prolonged uroflow pattern may be at higher risk of incomplete emptying.

An interrupted flow pattern can also be seen in patients with neurogenic lower urinary tract dysfunction and detrusor sphincter dyssynergia. Neurogenic patients who report stopping and starting of their urinary stream may be at higher risk of retention with OAB therapies, especially if their post-void residual is elevated. Considerable caution is warranted in performing a bladder neck suspension in this population.

Finally, the Qmax and uroflow pattern should not be interpreted in isolation. How uroflowmetry corresponds to the patient's symptoms and their PVR helps place the flow findings into clinical context.

Pad testing

Pad testing is a simple, noninvasive, and objective method for quantifying the severity of urinary incontinence. It's commonly used in research, but is not routinely performed in clinical practice. Pad testing in most cases does not change management.

The primary objective of pad testing is to determine the amount of urine leaked during a specified time and activity. The ICS has provided guidelines on performing a "1-hour pad test",[5] and the test is recommended by the FDA as an important endpoint when evaluating new treatments for female stress incontinence.

The test occupies a 1-hour time period in which a series of standardized activities are performed and fluid intake is controlled. The total amount of urine leaked during the time period is determined by weighing the final wet absorbent pad in grams and subtracting from it the pre-measured pad weight.

A change of pad weight of less than one gram is within experimental error and could be due to vaginal discharge, and as such the patient is considered dry. One gram weighed is equal to 1 mL, and therefore an increase in weight of the collection pad of 10 grams, for example, is equal to urinary incontinence of 10 mL.

Home pad tests lasting 24 and 48 hours are superior to the 1-hour test in detecting urinary incontinence but are less practical and more cumbersome. The collected pads must be stored in airtight containers to prevent evaporation prior to weighing. The 24-hour test is recognized as being most accurate because it's the most reproducible and has less chance of underestimating the severity of incontinence that sometimes plagues the 1-hour evaluation.

Although standard pad testing is rarely used in the evaluation of female incontinence, variations of pad testing are used in insensate incontinence, post-void dribbling, vaginal voiding, and vesicovaginal fistula evaluation. Coloration of the urine with oral Pyridium may increase the diagnostic value of the test.

More Sophisticated Urodynamic Assessment: Filling Cystometry

The principle aim of urodynamics is to reproduce the patient's urinary symptoms and to correlate them with the underlying physiologic measurements obtained in order to determine the pathophysiology of the symptoms.

Urodynamic testing simultaneously measures bladder pressure during bladder filling and emptying. It identifies the site of the lower urinary tract dysfunction to either the bladder, the bladder outlet/urethra, or both. Specific clinical questions are answered and, with the history and physical examination, a more precise diagnosis can be established. The severity of the condition may be determined and a treatment pathway planned.

Filling cystometry

Filling cystometry describes the urodynamic investigation of the filling phase of the micturition cycle. It utilizes real-time subtraction of the intraabdominal pressure from the intravesical pressure enabling identification of the detrusor pressure component.

Normally the bladder relaxes during urine storage and the outlet remains competently shut. During voiding, the detrusor forcefully contracts in a coordinated manner and the urethral sphincteric mechanism opens.

The filling phase starts when bladder filling commences and ends when the patient is given permission to void. Many advocate for a medium fill rate of 50 mL/min in nonneurogenic patients and 20 mL/min in those with neurogenic lower urinary tract dysfunction.

The four important components measured during filling cystometry include bladder sensation, detrusor activity, bladder compliance, and bladder capacity.

Bladder sensation

As recommended by the ICS, defined points of bladder sensation are routinely recorded during bladder filling. These include the volume in which the patient experiences their first sensation of bladder filling, the first desire to void, a strong desire to void, and the patient's maximum cystometric capacity (MCC). The MCC is the bladder volume in which the patient can no longer delay micturition and is given permission to voluntarily void.

Increased bladder sensation, once coined a hypersensitive bladder or sensory urgency, is when one or more of these sensory time points occur at low bladder volumes. Conversely, patients with reduced bladder sensation, or a hyposensitive one, have diminished sensation throughout filling and the sensations are registered at volumes higher than normal. Absent bladder sensation is when the individual has no bladder sensation during filling cystometry.

There are no "normal" values for these sensory time points and, given the subjectivity associated with their measurement, we recommend the following (Figure 10.1):

- Bladder sensation is important, but more so when it's clearly abnormal at either end of the sensory spectrum. A normal MCC is generally 400–600 mL, and most patients fall within this range. Some bladders are a bit more sensitive and experience urgency more than others, while some have delayed sensation of filling. But, all in all, there's minimal clinical significance to these mild variations.
- In contrast, for patients with a hypersensitive bladder with a MCC of less than approximately 300 mL, this is a positive and potentially clinically relevant finding. Feeling urgency and fullness at 120 mL is not normal and may impact treatment recommendations and outcome. Similarly, a large hyposensitive bladder of > 800 mL is an important urodynamic finding. Feeling the first sensation of bladder filling at 650 mL and leaking without awareness during detrusor overactivity is abnormal.

Figure 10.1 Bladder Sensation Spectrum

(A) Patients with normal bladder sensation generally have a MCC between 400-600 mL. (B) Patients with increased bladder sensation often have an MCC < 300 mL. (C) Patients with decreased bladder sensation typically have an MCC > 800 mL.

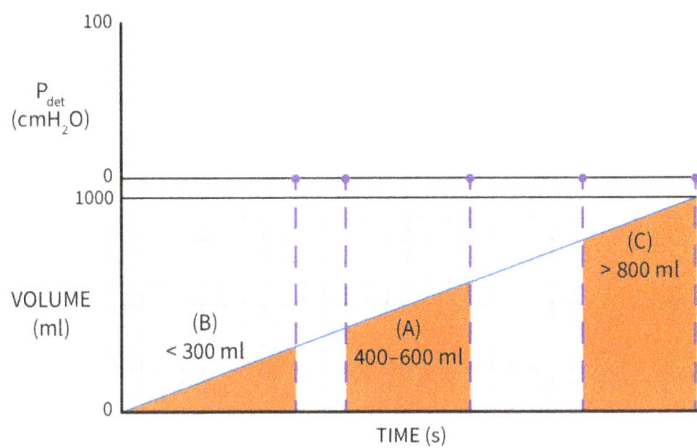

These urodynamic abnormalities at either end of the sensory spectrum should be taken into clinical consideration, as well as put into context with other urodynamic findings. Reduced or absent bladder sensation in a patient suspect of having a neurogenic bladder may be supportive of the diagnosis. A patient with stress urinary incontinence considering a sling and with a 950 mL hyposensitive and poorly contractile detrusor we believe is at higher risk of postoperative urinary retention. The same women with a hypersensitive bladder reporting urgency and fullness at 180 mL may experience significant urinary frequency following surgery.

Another bladder sensation that deserves attention during cystometry is the presence of urgency. A sudden desire to void should be recorded even in the absence of urgency incontinence. It's important to document at what volume the event occurs, and whether or not it is associated with a detrusor contraction.

The reporting of abdominal or suprapubic pain associated with bladder filling is critical. This may be an unexpected finding or an anticipated one based on clinical presentation. It may be the first clue that the patient has interstitial cystitis.

Patients with voiding dysfunction who are suspected of having bladder pain syndrome are carefully evaluated during cystometry. Paying attention to the patient's sensory awareness even to placing the catheter has implications. Often, those with IC/BPS will have discomfort with catheter insertion in addition to a hypersensitive bladder. We subjectively grade the patient's baseline discomfort after the catheter is placed and see if it worsens during filling cystometry. Worsening or lessening of the same pain during voiding is supportive of the diagnosis. Residual discomfort long after the test, with some patients calling the following day to report, is also seen in patients with bladder pain syndrome.

The art of urodynamics is understanding the nuances of the test and applying it to the individual patient. This applies to bladder sensation during filling. It is not just a box to check and to record, but potentially a subtle signal that is clinically significant. Paying attention to small details could avoid the dissatisfied experiences from a postoperative sling patient who, in retrospect, has a large capacity hyposensitive bladder and is now in urinary retention, or in the patient experiencing up-regulation of pelvic pain after a mesh sling.

Detrusor activity

During normal filling, the bladder is relaxed and compliant, with little to no change in bladder pressure, and without involuntary detrusor activity. Detrusor overactivity (DO) is a urodynamic observation characterized by the presence of involuntary detrusor contractions during filling cystometry, which may be spontaneous or provoked (Figure 10.2).

A number of patterns of detrusor overactivity have been described and deserve discussion. Phasic DO has a characteristic waveform pattern that is often repeated. Terminal DO is a single involuntary contraction occurring at cystometric capacity, which typically becomes increasingly uncomfortable and difficult to suppress. It's often high pressure and sustained relative to earlier contractions, and usually results in incontinence or permission to void.

Figure 10.2 Detrusor Overactivity

Detrusor overactivity (DO) is a urodynamic observation characterized by the presence of involuntary detrusor contractions during filling cystometry which may be spontaneous (A) or provoked (B).

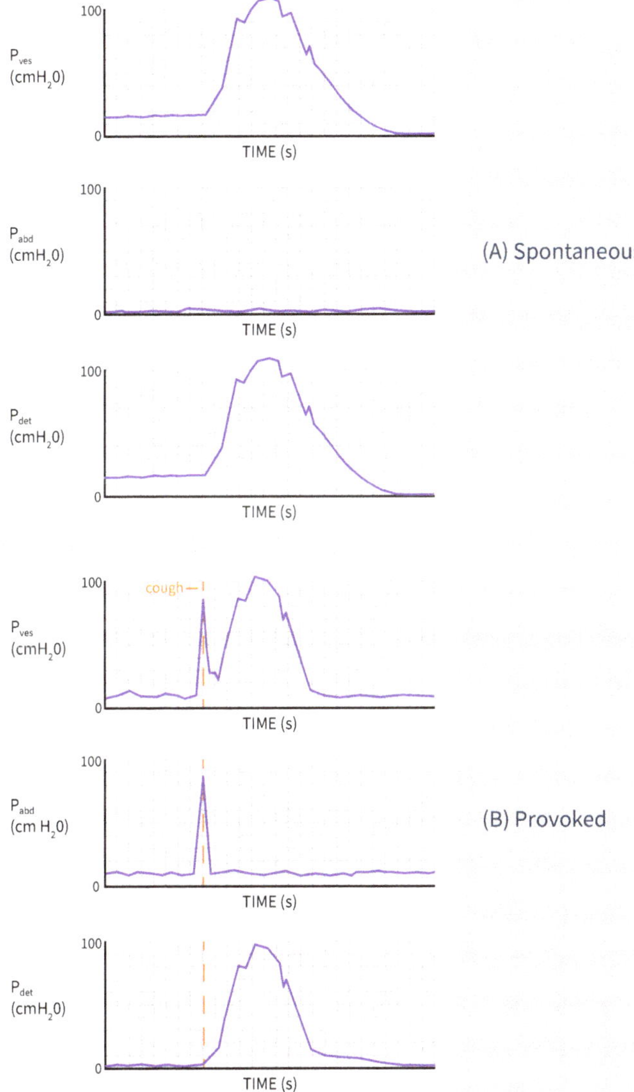

Idiopathic detrusor overactivity occurs when there is no defined etiology for the overactive detrusor. In contrast, neurogenic DO exists when the patient has an underlying neurologic condition resulting in their lower urinary tract dysfunction.

During cystometry a number of provocative maneuvers are recommended in order to unmask the presence of detrusor overactivity. These are especially important in those with storage symptoms, and who are not demonstrating DO. The techniques may be more effective at higher bladder volumes. Provocative maneuvers include coughing, rapid fill rates, running water, stepping, going from a sitting to standing position, and others. Enquiring from the patient what normally triggers their real-life urgency may be helpful in identifying which provocative step to use.

When DO is detected, a number of characterizations are important to document. The amplitude of the contraction, its duration, the volume at which it occurred, and the presence or absence of associated urgency or urgency incontinence should all be recorded. Whether the overactivity is spontaneous or provoked, the multiplicity and repetitiveness of DO should be noted.

Bladder Compliance

Bladder compliance describes the intrinsic ability of the bladder to increase in volume without a significant rise in detrusor pressure. It expresses the relationship between change in volume and change in pressure. The change in volume is divided by the change in detrusor pressure between two points, most commonly being the beginning of bladder filling and the patient's maximum cystometric capacity.

A number of calculations have been described, with a normal compliance being greater than 30–40 mL/cmH$_2$O. With each 30 to 40 mL increase in bladder volume there is less than 1 cmH$_2$O increase in detrusor pressure. Values less than 30 mL/cmH$_2$O represent hypo-compliance or poor compliance and are abnormal.

After decades of practice we seldom calculate bladder compliance. Instead, a quick look at the end filling detrusor pressure is a reasonable historic alternative. Generally speaking, a normal bladder capacity of

Figure 10.3 Loss of Bladder Compliance

The end filling pressure approaches zero in a normal bladder (A).
Patients with decreased bladder compliance (B) generally have an end
filling pressure greater than 10 cmH$_2$O.

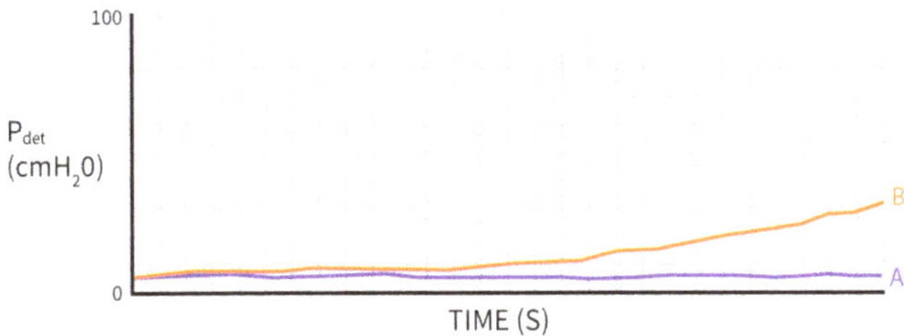

400–600 mL should have an end filling pressure approaching zero and
a value greater than 10 cmH$_2$O is likely abnormal. Clearly, an end filling
pressure of 20–40 cmH$_2$O or greater indicates significant bladder pathology and is clinically relevant (Figure 10.3). In contrast, a mild terminal
rise in detrusor pressure at high bladder volumes greater than 600 mL
is commonly seen and is normal.

Bladder compliance may be influenced by the non-physiologic
filling rate associated with urodynamics. Rapid filling may temporarily overwhelm the detrusor's elasticity, falsely elevating bladder
pressure. This is more commonly seen in patients with neurogenic
bladder and those with detrusor fibrosis. In order to minimize false
positives, it's recommended to wait approximately 30 seconds at the
end of filling before recording the end filling pressure. This short time
frame allows for muscle fiber accommodation and provides for a more
accurate measurement. Slower filling rates during cystometry may also
be effective.

Bladder capacity

The fourth component measured during filling cystometry is bladder
capacity. The maximum cystometric capacity (MCC) is the volume at
which the patient has a strong desire to void and feels that they can no
longer delay micturition. In contrast, the cystometric capacity is the

volume at the end of bladder filling when the permission to void is granted independent of bladder sensation. The two values are usually the same, but differ when bladder sensation is diminished or absent.

Regardless of definitions, the maximum capacity measured during cystometry is recorded. Importantly, the reason for stopping filling should be noted, and may include sensation of fullness, bladder pain, urinary incontinence, and bladder volume limit.

For example, an MCC defined by a strong desire to void is different from one due to pelvic pain in the same patient with voiding dysfunction. Some patients cannot be filled further because of urinary incontinence. In those with reduced bladder sensation, the capacity may be determined by stopping the study based on volume and not sensation. We generally stop filling beyond 900 mL since little additional information is gained and, conceptually, over filling might be detrimental to detrusor function. Having said that, men with known large bladder capacities are sometimes filled to very high volumes in order to adequately assess their voiding function. Ending filling prematurely may give a false assessment regarding their voiding capability.

Cystometric patterns

Cystometry provides an objective measure of the detrusor's storage capability. With little being referenced in the literature, we believe that there are favorable and unfavorable cystometric patterns or characteristics demonstrated during bladder filling. These favorable or unfavorable patterns to some degree help define the severity of the bladder's storage disorder, which could impact treatment recommendations and outcome.

For example, a single fleeting low pressure detrusor contraction occurring at 450 mL during cystometry and associated with mild urgency and no incontinence is different from multiple high-pressure contractions beginning early in bladder filling and associated with urgency incontinence or incontinence without awareness. Recognizing its unproven significance, the nature and severity of the bladder storage disorder appears profoundly different in these two circumstances.

Lacking established definitions, let us provide a number of representative cystometrograms that demonstrate unfavorable storage characteristics or a "bad bladder" (Figure 10.4).

Figure 10.4 Cystometry Patterns

Unfavorable storage characteristics

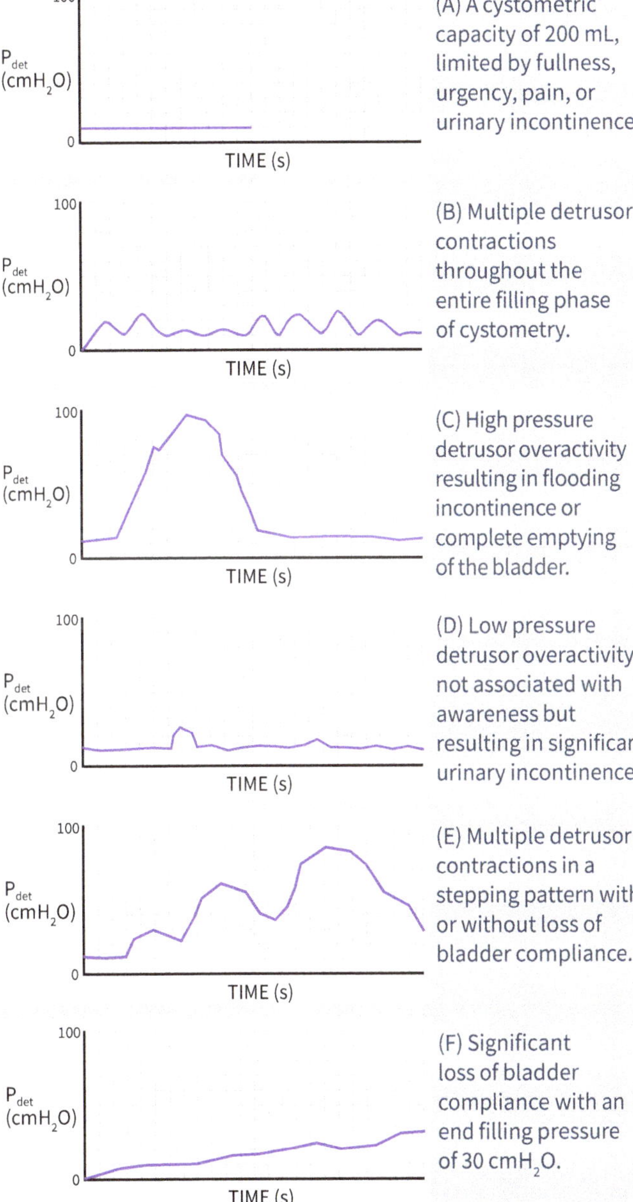

(A) A cystometric capacity of 200 mL, limited by fullness, urgency, pain, or urinary incontinence.

(B) Multiple detrusor contractions throughout the entire filling phase of cystometry.

(C) High pressure detrusor overactivity resulting in flooding incontinence or complete emptying of the bladder.

(D) Low pressure detrusor overactivity not associated with awareness but resulting in significant urinary incontinence.

(E) Multiple detrusor contractions in a stepping pattern with or without loss of bladder compliance.

(F) Significant loss of bladder compliance with an end filling pressure of 30 cmH₂O.

A comprehensive assessment

These cystometric patterns are common and have not been cherry-picked to make a point. Excluding decreased bladder compliance in females, these findings are regularly observed in patients with voiding dysfunction, especially those with storage symptoms.

The history and bladder diary are valuable in assessing bladder storage, but they do not predict cystometry. The only way to know the cystometric pattern is to do the study. Cystometry combined with the history and bladder diary observations provide the most comprehensive assessment of bladder storage, optimizing the provider's ability to recommend an effective treatment pathway.

> The history and bladder diary are valuable in assessing bladder storage but they do not predict cystometry.

As a general rule, the more you do urodynamics, the more you will realize that in many cases the voiding dysfunction is more of a bladder filling problem rather than a bladder outlet problem. Understanding this relationship will direct optimal therapy in patients that would be better served with an overactive bladder therapy versus a bladder neck suspension or a prostate procedure. Additionally, if surgical therapy is directed at the outlet as in SUI or BOO, knowledge of the nature of the bladder storage disorder beforehand is helpful.

The AUA/SUFU Adult Urodynamics Guidelines make a number of recommendations regarding the utilization of filling cystometry and multi-channel urodynamics in patients with voiding dysfunction.

Guidelines

According to the guidelines, cystometry may be performed in patients with stress incontinence and overactive bladder who are considering invasive, potentially morbid or irreversible treatments. They recommend that a complex cystometrogram should be performed during the initial evaluation of patients with relevant neurologic disorders and as part of their ongoing follow-up when appropriate. Other symptomatic neurogenic patients may also benefit from the evaluation. In male LUTS patients considering invasive therapy, cystometry may be performed when it's important to determine the presence of DO and other storage abnormalities.

We agree with the guideline statements but reflect upon their conservative nature. From a practical standpoint, the directives are vague and less beneficial based on their safe presentation. The "optionality" of using cystometry without providing more specific guidance does not instruct clinicians on how to use the test to help patients. Nor do they shed light on the use of cystometry in evaluating patients with more complicated voiding dysfunction, many of whom are only realized by doing the study.

In our modular series, we will thoroughly vet the use of cystometry in multiple patient populations and how it can be used to help recommend diagnosis to treatment pathways. We will illustrate how cystometry in combination with the history and other basic testing provides the most comprehensive assessment of bladder storage, and why the information is valuable, especially in those considering invasive, potentially morbid, or irreversible treatments.

Evaluation of Urethral Function

In order for adequate urine storage, the filling characteristics of the bladder must be favorable. In addition, a competent bladder neck and urethral sphincter mechanism are essential for urinary continence.

A normal urethral closure mechanism maintains its competence during increases in abdominal pressure. Urodynamic stress incontinence is the involuntary loss of urine during increases in intraabdominal pressure in the absence of a detrusor contraction. The presence of urodynamic SUI is an important component of the urodynamic assessment. Urethral characteristics ranging from a highly mobile urethra to an immobile one and the degree of intrinsic sphincter deficiency should be ascertained.

Two leak point pressures exist to assess urethral function during filling cytometry.

The abdominal leak point pressure (ALPP) is the intravesical pressure at which urine leakage occurs due to increased abdominal pressure in the absence of a detrusor contraction. It measures the ability of the bladder neck and urethral sphincter to resist increases in abdominal pressure, and is measured during coughing or a Valsalva maneuver.

- The cough leak point pressure (CLPP) is considered most clinically relevant but may be difficult to measure because of its rapidity.
- The Valsalva leak point pressure (VLPP) is slower and easier to record but some patients are unable to perform. Although the CLPP is generally thought to be superior in demonstrating SUI, both measures are often used in conjunction to provide maximum information.

The detrusor leak point pressure (DLPP) is used when evaluating patients with neurogenic lower urinary tract dysfunction, especially those with abnormal bladder compliance. The DLPP is the lowest detrusor pressure at which urine leakage occurs in the absence of either a detrusor contraction or increased intraabdominal pressure. Others will measure DLPP during overactive detrusor contractions in the same population of patients.

A DLPP of 40 cmH$_2$O is considered a reasonable cut-off for placing neurologically impaired patients such as those suffering from spina bifida at greater risk of upper tract damage secondary to high detrusor pressure. Having said that, renal deterioration has been noted to occur in patients with lower values.

Unfortunately, there is very little standardization as it pertains to measuring the VLPP and CLPP. Commonly measured at 200–300 mL, we record a number of values especially near bladder capacity. The pressure generated and the amount of urine lost is important. If present, LPP's should be measured with and without the pelvic organ prolapse reduced in search for varying results and to unmask occult SUI.

A guiding principle of urodynamics is attempting to replicate the patient's symptoms during the test. In SUI patients in whom objective evidence can't be demonstrated, a number of techniques are available. Some patients leak better while standing or after shifting their position. Others leak more readily at high bladder volumes. Removing the urethral catheter and repeating the stress test utilizing the rectal catheter measurement can unmask leakage in some women and men with SUI.

Urethral pressure measurement

A less commonly used measure of urethral function is the recording of urethral pressure. The urethral pressure is defined as the fluid pressure needed to just open a closed urethra. The maximum urethral closure pressure (MUCP) is the maximum difference between the urethral pressure and the intravesical pressure. It is generally accepted that a MUCP < 20 cmH$_2$O is in keeping with the presence of intrinsic sphincter deficiency.

The term intrinsic sphincter deficiency (ISD) was originally coined in the 1980s and was used to describe a severe form of SUI, equating it to an earlier term "type III stress urinary incontinence."[7] Although a precise definition of ISD is lacking, it is most commonly defined as an ALPP of less than 60 cmH_2O.

Guidelines

The guidelines state that clinicians making a diagnosis of urodynamic stress incontinence should assess urethral function.

The guideline is reasonably descriptive but less clear on how to use the measurement in clinical practice.

An estimation of the severity of urethral incompetence is important, as are other urethral characteristics. The urodynamic evaluation combined with the history and physical provides the most comprehensive assessment of urethral function, potentially influencing treatment pathways.

Remember, urodynamics is an art as much as a science, and the measurement of LPP is no exception. For example, a LPP of 20 cmH_2O is not a LPP of 140 in the same patient with SUI. Coughing repetitively and finally leaking a few drops at 60 cmH_2O is not flooding incontinence at the same pressure. A given LPP reproducible at 50–100 mL and throughout bladder filling is different from the same measure only demonstrated at near capacity.

In addition, a highly mobile urethra with significant rotational descent is different from one that only descends less than a cm. A fixed, short, scarred, stove-pipe urethra with a LPP of 10 cmH_2O is not a healthy appearing non-mobile one that leaks at high pressure.

It has been established that significantly low LPP's are associated with lower efficacy when managed surgically, and may influence choice of therapy. Recommending a retropubic or trans-obturator sling can be influenced by the urodynamic findings. Recommending urethral bulking agents may be based on LPP and the degree of hypermobility by some providers. A deeper dive into the clinical relevance of urethral function and how it potentially relates to therapy will be addressed in the SUI diagnosis to treatment module.

When noting the diagnosis of ISD or anatomical SUI, the terminology has less inter-provider relevance and meaning. The LPP, the amount of urine loss, at what volume, its ease of reproducibility, and the degree of urethral mobility are more clinically important and should be recorded.

Table 11.1: Urethral characteristics
Urethral mobility
- Degree of hypermobility
- Fixed urethra
Abdominal leak point pressure (cough and/or Valsalva)
- LPP recorded
- At what volume
- Amount of urine loss
Urethral pressure measurement
- Maximum urethral closure pressure

Pressure Flow Studies

Once the storage characteristics of the detrusor and the competence of the urethral sphincter have been established, the voiding phase of cystometry begins by instructing the patient to voluntarily void. The voiding phase evaluates the detrusor's ability to contract in a coordinated fashion and the urethra to relax simultaneously. During pressure flow studies the detrusor pressure and uroflow parameters are captured and voiding efficiency is assessed.

Bladder outlet obstruction (BOO) is a urodynamic diagnosis characterized by an increased detrusor pressure and reduced flow rate. Two detrusor pressures are available for the analysis.

The maximum detrusor pressure, $P_{det}max$, is the maximum value measured at the peak of the voiding pressure curve. It is clinically relevant in determining the presence of bladder outlet obstruction or a poorly contractile bladder. The pressure at maximum flow, $P_{det}@Qmax$, is the detrusor pressure recorded during maximum flow and is also helpful in assessing voiding function. Normal maximum detrusor pressure varies with age and gender but generally ranges between 25 and 50 cmH$_2$O.

A normal maximum urinary flow rate (Qmax) in women is greater than 30 to 35 mL/sec, but lower rates are commonly observed in women reporting normal voiding. Many women can only generate weak detrusor contractions but void efficiently by simultaneously relaxing their pelvic floor.

Young men under 40 years of age generally have a Qmax of greater than 25 mL/sec. A flow rate of greater than 15 mL/sec is considered normal in men over 60 years.

In men, an abnormally high voiding pressure accompanied by a weak or prolonged urinary flow is characteristic of obstruction. Many experts regard a P_{det}max greater than 60 cmH$_2$O associated with a Qmax of less than 10 mL/sec to be diagnostic. A P_{det}max of > 100 cmH$_2$O regardless of Qmax also signifies obstruction.

In many cases the presence of BOO is more equivocal. For instance, when the detrusor pressure can forcibly overcome obstruction leading to a high pressure but normal flow situation. In others, some patients with normal pressure and low flow rates are also obstructed. Their detrusor has not yet accommodated to the obstruction, or it has partially failed and unable to produce high pressure. The result is normal or low pressure voiding in combination with low flow.

As an aid in determining if BOO is present, the ICS pressure/flow nomogram can be used to calculate the bladder outflow obstruction index (BOOI).[8] It and other well-established nomograms categorize patients as being obstructed, unobstructed, or equivocal. Modern urodynamic software automatically plots the nomograms, or they can be easily calculated utilizing a simple formula (Figure 12.1).

Figure 12.1: Bladder outflow obstruction index (BOOI)

$$BOOI = P_{det}@Qmax - (2x\ Qmax)$$

BOOI < 20 = unobstructed

BOOI > 40 = obstructed

BOOI 20–40 = equivocal

In addition to diagnosing obstruction, pressure flow studies identify the presence of detrusor underactivity in patients with flow symptoms. A low detrusor pressure or a poorly sustained detrusor contraction in combination with a low flow rate is representative of detrusor underactivity. An acontractile detrusor dose not contract during voiding, and both findings can be non-neurogenic or neurogenic in origin.

It is also important to note that not all BOO is due to the prostate. Functional obstruction results from inadequate or variable relaxation of the urethral sphincter and pelvic floor. In addition to a slow stream, the flow may also be intermittent. Pelvic floor dyssynergia occurs in non-neurologic patients and sometimes begins early in childhood.

The term detrusor sphincter dyssynergia is used to describe the dyscoordination between the detrusor and rhabdosphincter during voiding in patients with a neurological abnormality. In addition to having abnormal flow, the patients may also have high voiding pressure that can threaten renal health.

An interesting population of men with lower urinary tract symptoms have primary bladder neck obstruction. During voiding, the bladder neck smooth muscle fails to adequately open and these often younger patients can be highly symptomatic. The role of video-urodynamics in establishing a diagnosis of bladder neck dyssynergia will be vetted in one of the diagnosis to treatment pathway modules.

An eyeball approach

A number of numeric definitions of BOO exist, but a simple eyeball approach is adequate in making the diagnosis in most cases. The observation of the presence of a well sustained high pressure detrusor contraction associated with a poor, intermittent, or prolonged flow is usually sufficient.

We recommend to note three aspects of the pressure flow relationship during its analysis: the maximum voiding pressure, the Qmax generated, and, importantly, whether or not the detrusor contraction is well sustained (Figure 12.2).

When interpreting pressure flow, it's important to consider what is normal in the same aged patient and apply the findings to the clinical presentation. Ask yourself if you think the voiding findings represent obstruction in context to the circumstance, and whether or not it's clinically relevant. Pay less attention to the actual numbers and focus more on the entire voiding picture.

For example, a symptomatic 52 year-old man with a normal, well sustained detrusor contraction of 30 cmH$_2$O associated with a Qmax of 6 mL/sec is partially obstructed. His flow should be perfectly normal with his detrusor capability. In the same circumstance, a poorly sustained fleeting contraction of 30 cmH$_2$O, lasting only a few seconds and with the same Qmax, represents a weak detrusor and not BOO. Especially in the case of men, detrusor contractions must be well sustained in order to empty efficiently.

Figure 12.2 Pressure Flow Studies

An eyeball approach to evaluate the pressure flow:

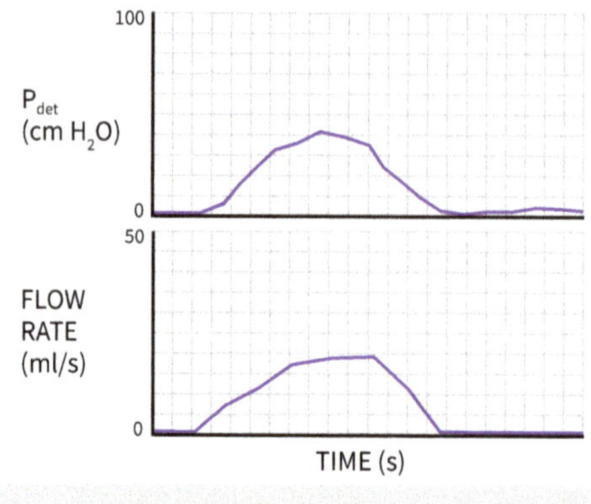

(A) Patient generates a well sustained normal voiding pressure with a normal flow.

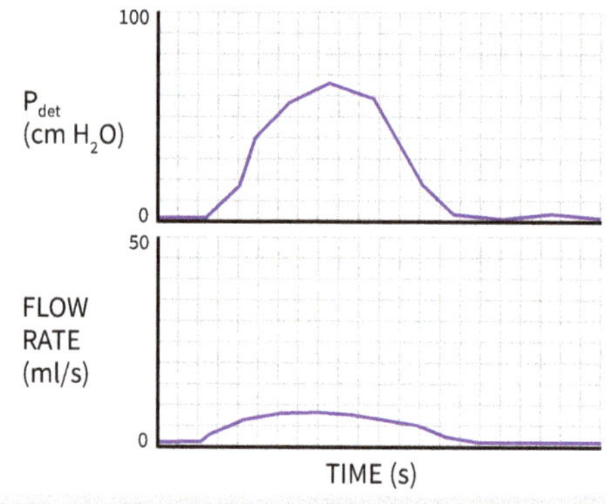

(B) Patient generates a well sustained high voiding pressure with a low flow.

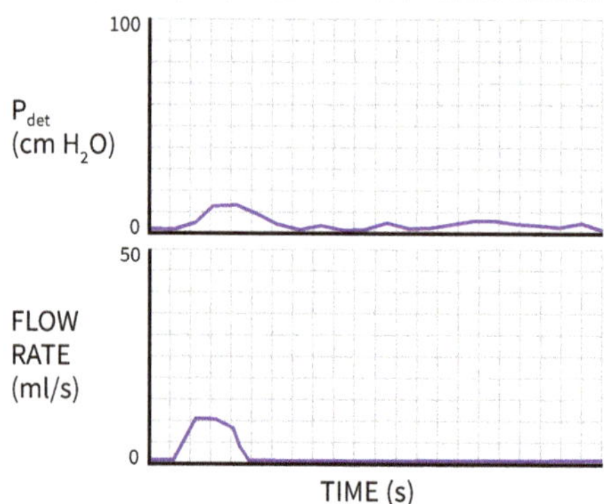

(C) Patient generates a poorly sustained low pressure detrusor contraction and has a low flow.

Similarly, an elderly man generating a well sustained detrusor contraction of 20 cmH$_2$O and who is in urinary retention is obstructed. He should be able to void even with the less than normal voiding pressure. The same pressure in the same man voiding spontaneously with a reduced flow is not obstructed. His flow symptoms are from a weakened detrusor, especially if the contraction is poorly sustained.

Finally, when evaluating pressure flow, the void must be voluntary. When patients have terminal detrusor overactivity and void, they are not voiding voluntarily but rather reflexively voiding. Voiding off the top of such an involuntary terminal contraction is not adequate for pressure flow analysis. The patient must be refilled and asked to void voluntarily, usually at a lower volume.

A number of numeric definitions of BOO exist but a simple eyeball approach is adequate in making the diagnosis in most cases. The observation of the presence of a well sustained high pressure detrusor contraction associated with a poor, intermittent, or prolonged flow is usually sufficient.

UroCuff™ testing

More recently, a non-invasive bladder test has been developed to effectively measure pressure flow. The CT3000 UroCuff™ is a simple, rapid test that readily differentiates between bladder outlet obstruction and poor bladder contractility in men with lower urinary tract symptoms (Figure 12.3). The device is fitted to the penis and the patient is asked to voluntarily void into a uroflowmeter.

Figure 12.3

The CT3000 UroCuff™ is a simple, rapid test that readily differentiates between bladder outlet obstruction and poor bladder contractility in men with LUTS.

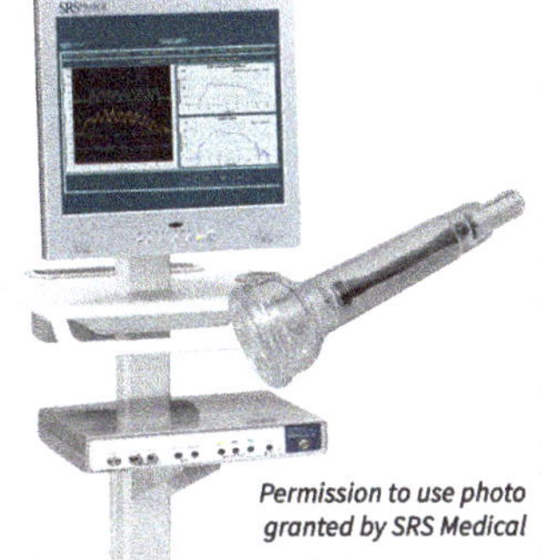

Permission to use photo granted by SRS Medical

The highest voiding pressure at flow interruption ($P_{CuffInt}$) and Qmax are measured and plotted on a modified version of the ICS nomogram. Using the isovolumetric bladder pressure and maximum flow, the patients are categorized as being obstructed, not obstructed, high pressure high flow, or low pressure low flow (Figure 12.4).

Figure 12.4

Using a modified version of the ICS nomogram, UroCuff™ categorizes patients as being obstructed, not obstructed, high pressure high flow, and low pressure low flow.

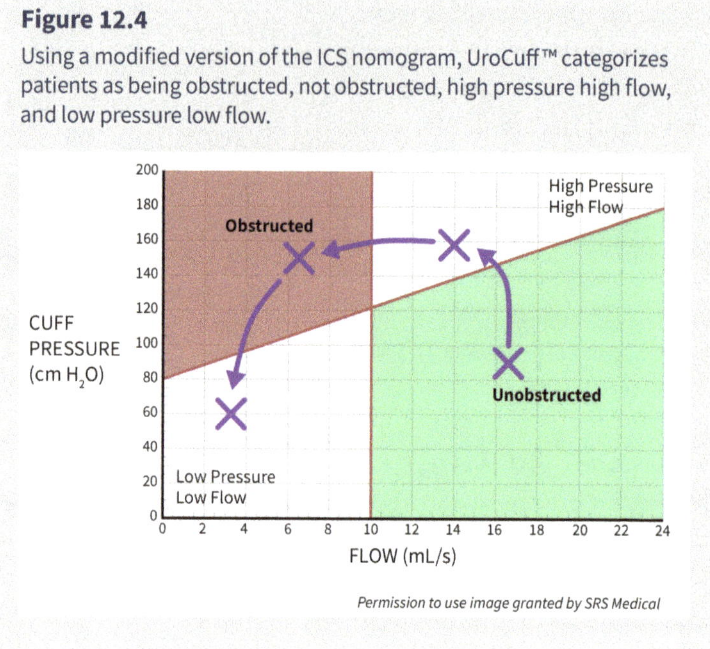

Permission to use image granted by SRS Medical

The correlation of this non-invasive pressure flow analysis with catheter-based urodynamics is excellent, and arguably may be a more natural representation of voiding. In addition to identifying patients with BOO, it is an excellent way to follow voiding pressures in male LUTS patients who are being managed conservatively. Objectively demonstrating increasing BOO or a failing detrusor over time may alter treatment recommendations in many patients. The liberal use of this device in clinical practice will likely shed light on the natural history of voiding pressure in men with LUTS and impact future therapy.

The simplicity, cost-effectiveness, and non-invasive nature of UroCuff™ makes it attractive and it's a positive step forward for providers in evaluating symptomatic men. Having said that, the test does not replace the liberal utilization of formal urodynamics in this population, as it does not assess the bladder's storage characteristics. We predict that a hybrid approach adopting both urodynamics and UroCuff™ testing into clinical practice will become popular.

The Adult Urodynamic Guidelines make a number of directive statements regarding the use of pressure flow studies in women and men with voiding dysfunction.

Guidelines

Clinicians may perform pressure flow studies in females who report a new onset of urgency incontinence following a bladder neck suspension to evaluate for bladder outlet obstruction.

In women with significant elevations in PVR, urinary retention or definite alterations in voiding symptoms following an anti-incontinence procedure, these findings strongly imply BOO, and urodynamics may not be necessary before intervention.

The guidelines also state that clinicians may perform pressure flow studies in females with lower urinary tract symptoms when it's important to determine if obstruction is present.

Pressure flow studies should be performed during the initial urological evaluation of male and female patients with relevant neurological conditions and as part of their ongoing follow-up when appropriate. Symptomatic others with neurologic disorders should be considered especially those with an elevated postvoid residual.

The guidelines recommend that pressure flow studies in symptomatic men should be performed when it's important to determine if urodynamic obstruction is present in men with LUTS, particularly when invasive, potentially morbid or irreversible treatments are considered.

We approve of the guideline directives but would like to make a number of comments.

Pressure flow studies are less definitive and clinically relevant in women versus men, but still play an important role. Those with de novo obstructive or storage symptoms following a bladder neck suspension should be studied. The diagnosis of obstruction can be difficult and urodynamic assessment is warranted. Making the diagnosis can be even more challenging when the initial surgery was done years prior. The utilization of pressure flow and cystometry in this challenging population will be detailed in one of the diagnosis to treatment pathway modules.

The guidelines directing clinicians to perform pressure flow studies in women with LUTS when it is important to determine if obstruction is present is vague and lacks clinical relevance.

Instead, we recommend pressure flow in women with bothersome obstructive urinary symptoms who fail alpha-blockers and physical therapy and who are considering neuromodulation. Sacral nerve modulation is much more effective in women with pelvic floor dyssynergia than in those with a poorly contractile detrusor.

Pressure flow is part of the clinical assessment of women with SUI who are considering a bladder neck suspension. The presence of a poorly contractile detrusor or significant pelvic floor dyssynergia likely increase the risk of retention and should be realized prior to surgery.

Male and female patients with relevant neurological conditions are at risk of developing renal deterioration secondary to high bladder pressure during both filling and emptying. We agree that the majority should be evaluated with filling and pressure flow cystometry in order to recommend their bladder management program and long-term surveillance.

We agree with the guidelines recommending pressure flow studies in symptomatic men when it's important to determine if urodynamic obstruction is present, particularly when invasive, potentially morbid, or irreversible treatments are considered.

Evidence has shown that surgical results are superior in men who are urodynamically obstructed. Having said that, the phraseology of "when it's important" is interesting and deserves discussion.

When would it not be important to determine whether or not a male LUTS patient with flow symptoms was obstructed when considering a prostatectomy or invasive procedure? The only way to know if he has a poorly contractile or acontractile bladder and is likely not to benefit from the procedure is to do the study. Hence nearly all patients considering surgery should be evaluated.

Although the guideline statements are reasonable, we take a much more bullish approach to urodynamics and pressure flow studies. Proceeding with invasive prostate-directed therapy without filling and voiding cystometry in most patients does not allow for optimal patient/physician shared decision making. We will highlight the use of these tests in the BPH diagnosis to treatment pathway module.

Electromyography

Electromyography (EMG) is the study of the bioelectric potentials generated by depolarization of skeletal muscle. An excitatory impulse in the motor neuron causes muscle fibers to contract, the sum of which is called the motor unit action potential (MUCP). The resulting EMG waveform is simultaneously portrayed on the urodynamic monitor or strip chart during filling and pressure flow cystometry.

Surface electrodes record the total electrical output from the muscles of the pelvic floor, external urinary sphincter, and external anal sphincter. Patches placed next to the anus are most commonly used and provide a fair representation of pelvic floor and urethral sphincter activity. The location allows for simple application, and dislodgement is less common.

Unlike concentric needle electrodes, surface patches don't measure individual MUAPs, but are more comfortable and less invasive. The practical application of EMG involves determination of whether the perineal muscles are relaxed or contracting during bladder filling and emptying. Most importantly, it determines whether the perineal activity is coordinated or uncoordinated with detrusor contractions.

During bladder filling, there's a normal progressive increase in EMG activity referred to as recruitment. Just prior to voiding, the urethral sphincter relaxes with a corresponding silencing of EMG activity. The reduced excitatory activity should persist throughout micturition (Figure 13.1).

Figure 13.1 Normal recruitment and relaxation during voiding

Normal recruitment of increased EMG activity as the bladder fills. EMG activity silences or lessens during micturition.

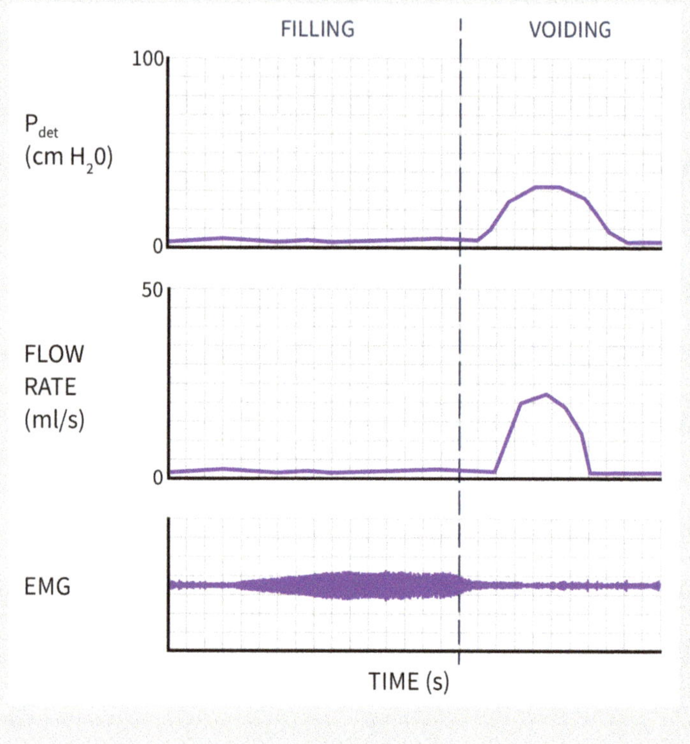

Persistent or increased EMG activity during voiding can be due to a number of factors. First, it's normal that complete electrical silence does not occur in many patients, and increased activity can be secondary to movement or straining. The straining artifact of increased EMG activity associated with increases in abdominal pressure during voiding has been well described (Figure 13.2).

Figure 13.2 Straining or movement artifact

The "straining artifact" of increased EMG activity associated with increases in abdominal pressure during voiding.

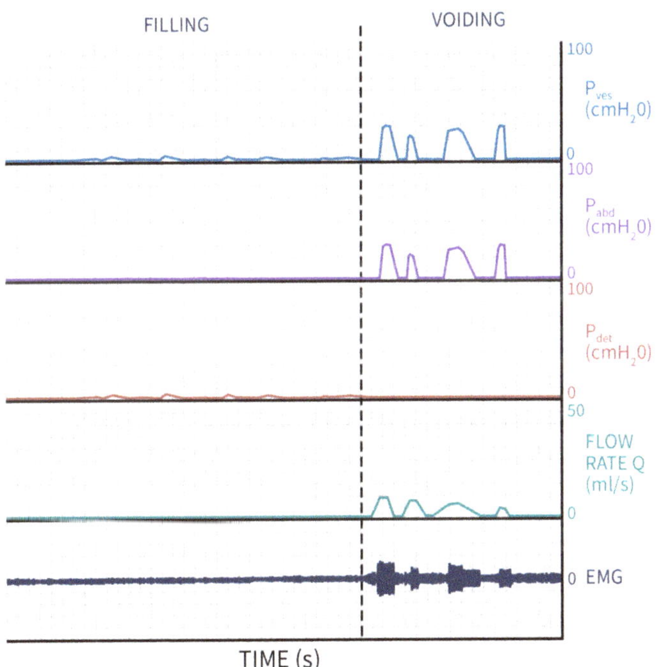

Pelvic floor dyssynergia is frequent in both symptomatic and asymptomatic patients. Women commonly don't naturally relax their pelvic floor and urethral sphincter during voiding, in many cases dating back to childhood. Many others with bladder pain syndrome demonstrate impressive increased EMG activity while voiding due to pelvic floor dyssynergia (Figure 13.3).

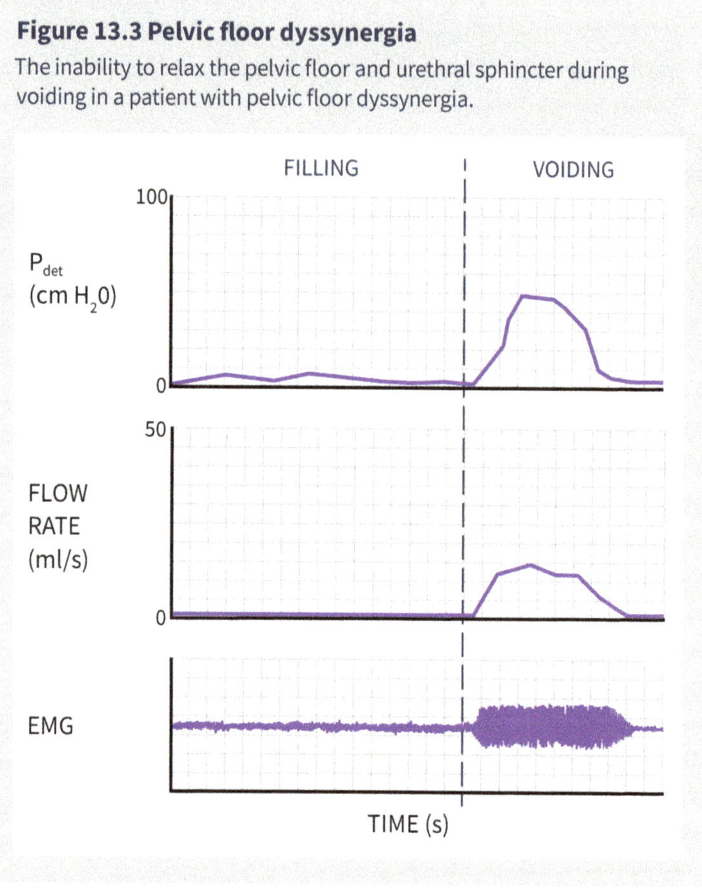

Figure 13.3 Pelvic floor dyssynergia
The inability to relax the pelvic floor and urethral sphincter during voiding in a patient with pelvic floor dyssynergia.

In contrast, pseudodyssynergia is the normal voluntary contraction of the external urethral sphincter and pelvic floor muscles in response to an involuntary detrusor contraction in an attempt to prevent urgency incontinence. With varying ability to do so, patients may abate the contraction and avoid urinary leakage (Figure 13.4).

Figure 13.4 Pseudodyssynergia

Pseudodyssynergia is the normal voluntary contraction of the external urethral sphincter and pelvic floor in response to an involuntary detrusor contraction in an attempt to prevent urgency incontinence. The EMG silences during voiding.

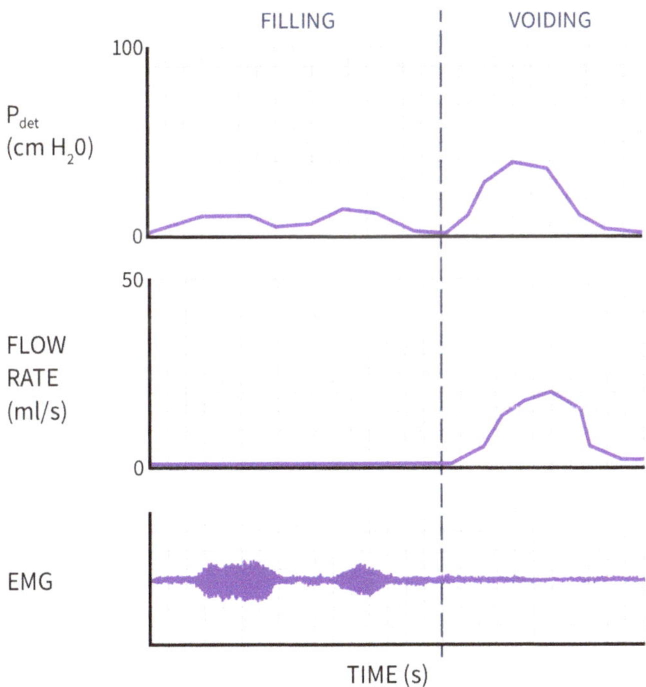

As noted, true detrusor sphincter dyssynergia (DSD) occurs only in patients with neurological disorders and is pathognomonic for the diagnosis of neurogenic bladder dysfunction. In addition to causing voiding symptoms and obstruction, the development of high voiding pressures may threaten renal health.

The guideline statements regarding the measurement of EMG during urodynamics are limited to voiding dysfunction in patients with neurological disease.

Guidelines

Physicians should perform EMG in combination with CMG with or without pressure flow in patients with relevant neurologic disease at risk of neurogenic bladder, in patients with other neurologic disease and elevated PVR or in patients with urinary symptoms.

We agree with these directives but would like to make additional comments and recommendations.

As part of the voiding phase assessment, EMG testing is important in evaluating patients with various lower urinary tract symptoms since it may have diagnostic and therapeutic relevance.

Many men and women with bladder outlet obstruction and reduced or intermittent flow have underlying pelvic floor dyssynergia, and the diagnosis helps direct effective therapy. Similarly, the causal or contributory relationship of dyssynergia with OAB is important to realize and treating it can be beneficial. Although unproven, women considering a sling and who have symptomatic pelvic floor dysfunction could experience more voiding complaints postoperatively.

The presence of increased EMG activity during voiding may also support the diagnosis of other underlying pathology. For instance, in an undiagnosed patient reporting worsening symptoms following lumbar disc surgery or another with vague neurologic symptoms, the presence of DSD may aid in the diagnosis of neurogenic bladder dysfunction. As noted, the presence of pelvic floor dyssynergia in patients suspect of having bladder pain syndrome may be supportive.

The guidelines express that a limitation of EMG testing is its non-specific nature and that artifacts in EMG activity are common. Importantly, EMG should be taken into context with the patient's presenting complaint, as well as with filling cystometry and pressure flow in order to make the most accurate diagnosis. When available, correlation of the EMG activity with the presence of fluoroscopic narrowing of the urethra can augment its diagnostic potential.

The art of EMG testing is knowing when EMG matters. In the majority of voiding dysfunction patients, the EMG has little to no clinical consequence. In others, such a subtle sign or positive finding can have diagnostic and therapeutic relevance.

Video-Urodynamics

Video-urodynamics is the simultaneous fluoroscopic imaging of the bladder and urethra during filling and voiding cystometry. It aids clinicians in detecting and understanding underlying pathology, and is beneficial in select patients.

Figure 14. 1 Video-urodynamics lab

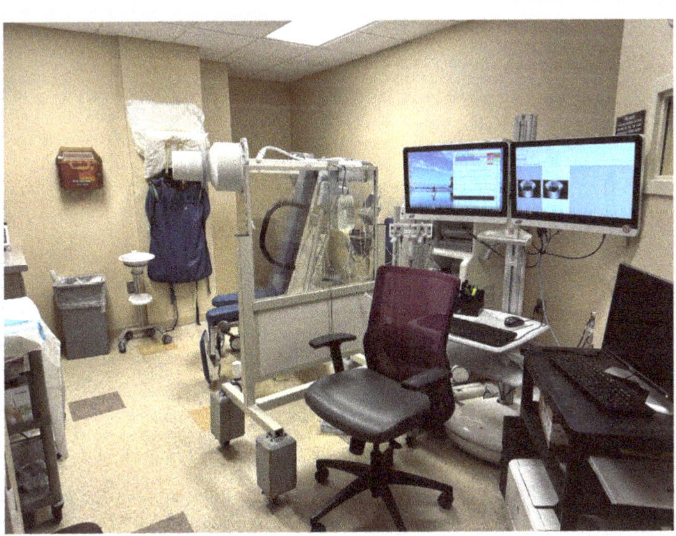

We agree with the guidelines that make a few directive statements regarding the use of video-urodynamics in clinical practice. Having said that, we use fluoroscopy in all patients, and find it to be clinically beneficial. Many abnormalities are not predictable and would be missed otherwise.

Guidelines

Clinicians may perform video-urodynamics in properly selected LUTS patients to localize the level of obstruction, particularly the diagnosis of primary bladder neck obstruction.

When available, clinicians may perform fluoroscopy at the time of urodynamics (video-urodynamics) in patients with relevant neurologic disease at risk of neurogenic bladder, in patients with other neurologic disease and elevated PVR or in patients with urinary symptoms.

Fluoroscopy: BPH

Fluoroscopy during voiding helps identify the location of obstruction. An enlarged prostate may demonstrate a reduced caliber of the prostatic urethra and an indentation of the bladder base (Figure 14.2). With larger glands, the length of the prostatic urethra may appear lengthened.

Figure 14.2 Fluoroscopy: BPH

Elderly male with high pressure low flow bladder outlet obstruction secondary to BPH. The bladder base is elevated from an enlarged prostate.

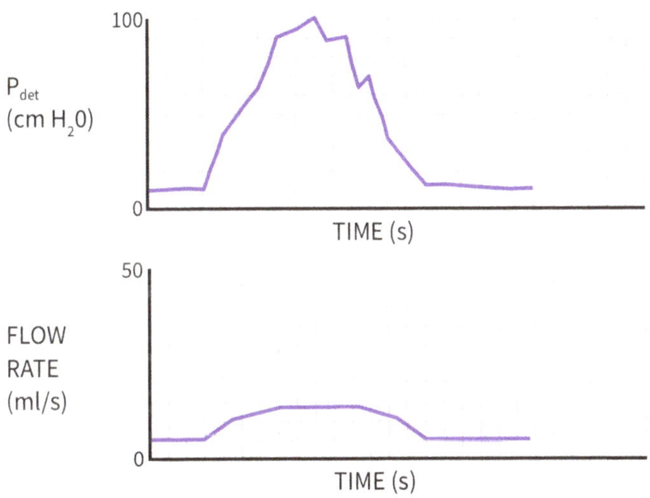

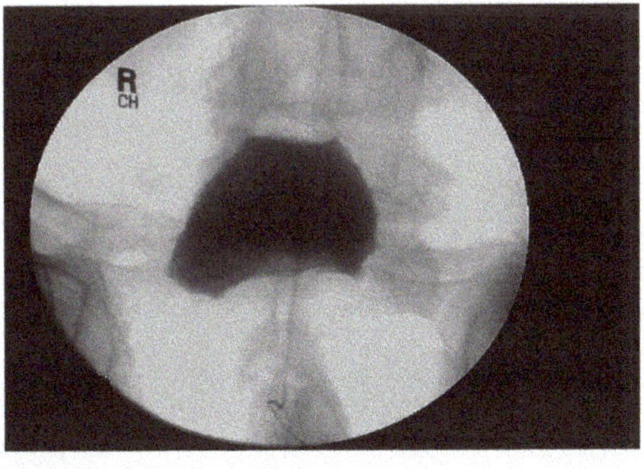

Fluoroscopy: Primary bladder neck obstruction

Primary bladder neck obstruction is a video-urodynamic diagnosis that is usually made in younger men. During voluntary voiding there is a delay or failure of the bladder neck to open. The hallmark of primary bladder neck obstruction is high pressure low flow voiding with radiographic evidence of obstruction at the bladder neck and simultaneous relaxation of the distal urethral sphincter (Figure 14.3).

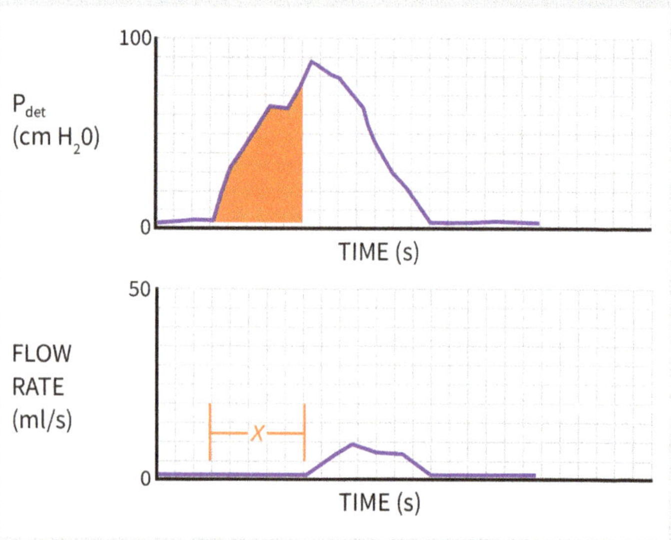

Figure 14.3 Fluoroscopy: Bladder neck obstruction
The patient has bladder neck dyssynergia. There is a delay in the opening time (X). The bladder contracts but there is initially no flow due to failure of the bladder neck to open.

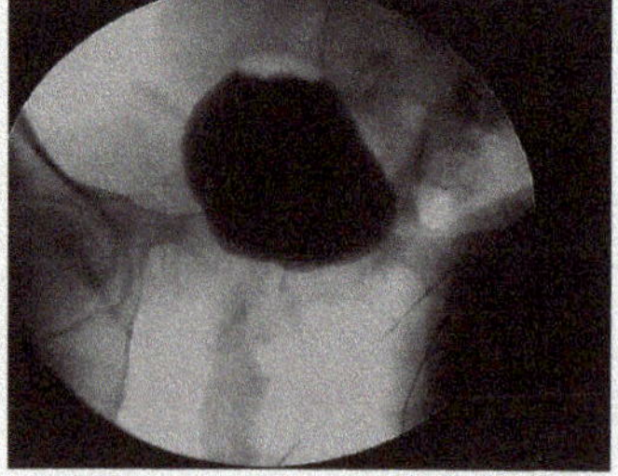

He has high pressure low flow voiding with radiographic evidence of bladder neck obstruction.

Fluoroscopy: Pelvic floor dyssynergia (spinning top)

Pelvic floor dyssynergia is depicted by obstruction of contrast at the level of the striated external sphincter. More common in women, the urethra may develop a 'spinning top' appearance due to widening of the posterior urethra from chronic high pressure trapping of urine above the level of the obstruction (Figure 14.4). Pelvic floor dyssynergia is differentiated from DSD by the absence of a neurologic diagnosis.

Figure 14.4 Fluoroscopy: Pelvic floor dyssynergia

Fluoroscopic image of female patient with pelvic floor dyssynergia. The contrast is obstructed at the level of the external sphincter and she has a mild 'spinning top' deformity of the proximal urethra.

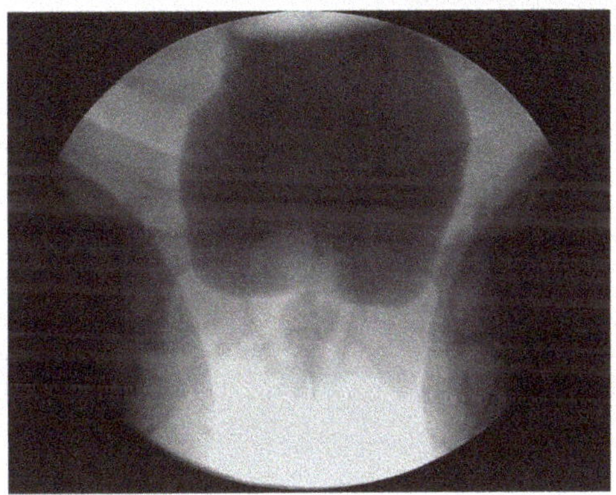

Fluoroscopy: Anatomic abnormalities

Chronic fluoroscopic changes in the bladder, such as trabeculation, diverticula, and vesicoureteral reflux may be seen in patients with high filling and voiding pressures. The presence and grade of reflux and the urodynamic parameters that are occurring simultaneously should be noted.

Although unproven, bladder trabeculation may also result from repetitive detrusor overactivity during bladder filling. Impressive chronic bladder changes may be a predictor of persistent storage symptoms in patients managed with a sling or invasive prostate-directed therapy for mixed symptoms.

Fluoroscopy provides an excellent assessment of the post-void residual urine volume. Patients with elevated residuals following voiding cystometry should be asked to double void catheter free in private, and then have their PVR rechecked with fluoroscopy. Video is also an effective way to estimate residual urine volumes in spinal cord patients who empty by reflex voiding.

A number of additional anatomic abnormalities can be identified radiographically. The presence of a vesicovaginal fistula or urethral diverticulum can be diagnosed and a filling defect may suggest the presence of a bladder stone or malignancy.

Fluoroscopy: Neurogenic bladder dysfunction

We agree with the guidelines that video-urodynamics improves the diagnostic evaluation of patients with neurological disease. It may also provide evidence of neurogenic bladder in those with risk factors but no formal diagnosis. A poorly compliant heavily trabeculated detrusor and the presence of a Christmas tree shaped bladder is highly suggestive of a neurologic etiology (Figure 14.5). Detrusor sphincter dyssynergia demonstrated by EMG activity and contrast obstructed at the level of the distal sphincter is pathognomonic.

Figure 14.5 Fluoroscopy: Neurogenic bladder dysfunction
Male patient with Christmas tree shaped neurogenic bladder. Patient has had previous spinal surgery.

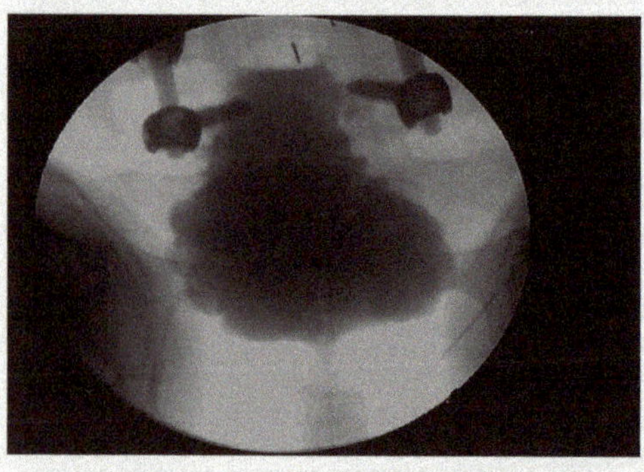

Fluoroscopy: Stress incontinence and prolapse

In addition to evaluating obstruction and neurogenic bladder, fluoroscopy is helpful in assessing female patients with SUI and prolapse.

With the patient standing or sitting, the position of the bladder neck at rest and during increases in abdominal pressure can be visualized (Figure 14.6). Supine patients with an apparent immobile urethra on pelvic examination may demonstrate bladder neck descensus while sitting during fluoroscopy. Similarly, an initial small cystocele in a symptomatic patient may appear radiographically larger supporting its clinical relevance.

14.6: Fluoroscopy: Hypermobility of the bladder neck in a women with stress urinary incontinence.

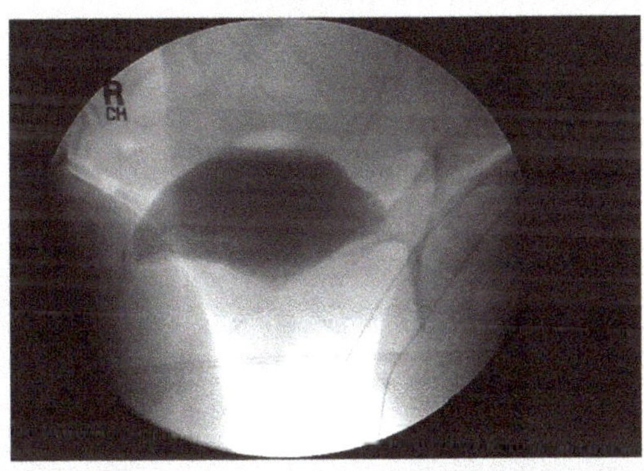

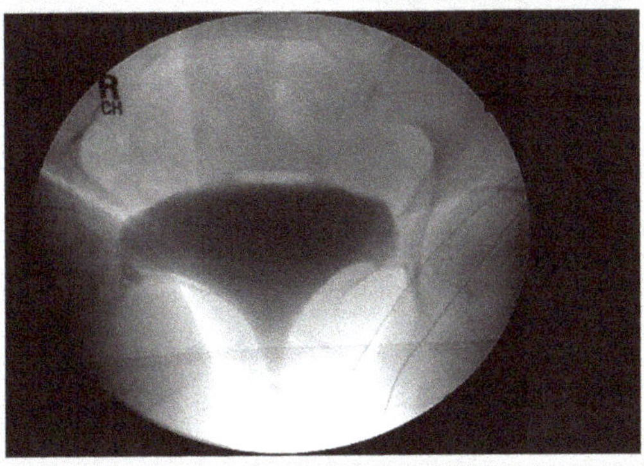

Urinary leakage can be visualized fluoroscopically, but it may need to be higher volume in order to be detected. Direct inspection of the vaginal introitus and the patient reporting when they leaked is generally recommended in order to obtain an accurate leak point pressure.

Beaking of the bladder neck during increases in abdominal pressure is commonly demonstrated in continent women and is considered normal. This should be differentiated from the rectangular-shaped incompetent bladder neck sometimes visualized in patients with ISD (Figure 14.7).

Figure 14.7 Fluoroscopy: Evaluation of the bladder neck

(A) Beaking: Beaking of the bladder neck is a normal finding commonly seen in continent women.

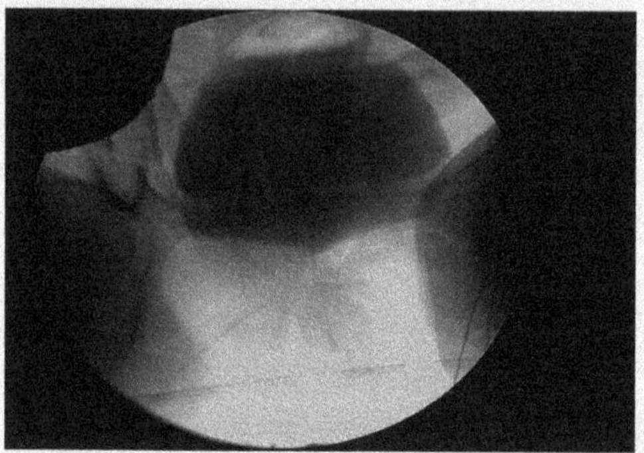

(B) Rectangular: A "rectangular-shaped" incompetent bladder neck is in keeping with the diagnosis of ISD.

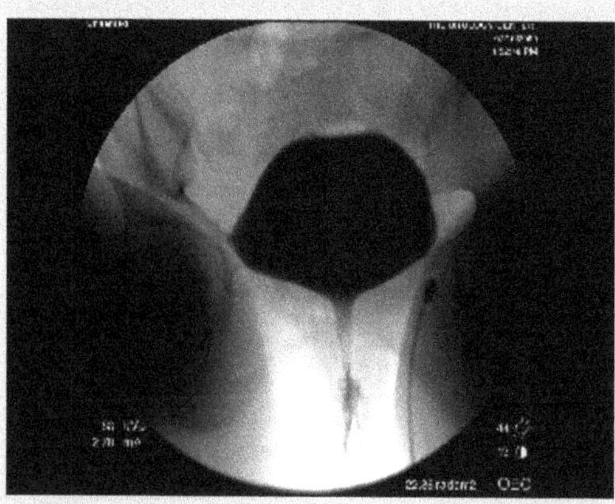

When using a fluoroscopy table with the patient in the semi-lateral oblique position, the bladder neck can be differentiated from a dependent cystocele. The severity of the prolapse and its functional significance can also be evaluated. For larger cystoceles associated with flow symptoms or elevated residuals, the voiding phase should be performed with and without the prolapse reduced and demonstrated fluoroscopically. Elevated residuals secondary to prolapse may normalize following cystocele reduction.

With the widespread use of fluoroscopy chairs, the differentiation between the bladder neck and a cystocele can be more challenging giving false positives regarding the degree of bladder neck hypermobility. A difference in the cystogram contrast intensity visualized with anterior posterior imaging is helpful in differentiating the two (Figure 14.8).

Figure 14.8 Fluroscopy: The differentiation of the bladder neck versus a cystocele

The anterior posterior imaging of the bladder differentiates a "lighter gray" cystocele from the "darker bladder and bladder neck". There is less contrast in the dependent cystocele versus the bladder.

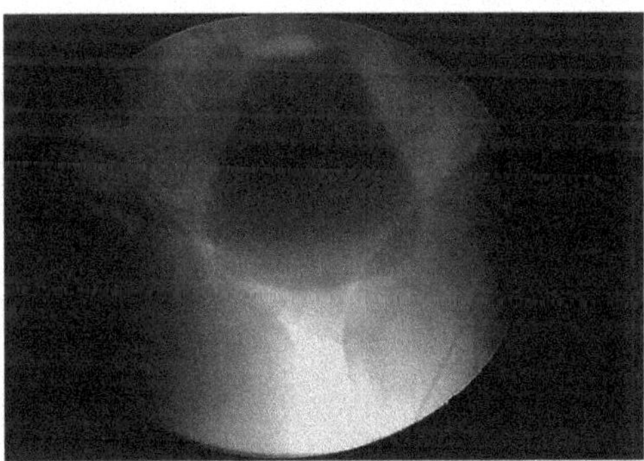

Video-urodynamics is beneficial in the evaluation of many patients with voiding dysfunction, but its cost and required resources makes it less practical to most physicians. Having said that, urodynamics plus video is better than urodynamics alone, and, for those with busy and extensive voiding dysfunction practices, they may consider the investment worthwhile.

Cystoscopy

Urologists are aware of the benefit and indications for cystoscopy which is liberally performed in daily practice. Cystoscopy provides an anatomic assessment of the bladder and urethra, and plays an important role in many patients with voiding dysfunction.

Patients with hematuria and those suspect of having an intravesical cause of their urinary symptoms should be evaluated. The presence of bladder or urethral mesh, bladder calculi or carcinoma, diverticula, genitourinary fistula, or local radiation changes are all confirmed by endoscopy (Figure 15.1).

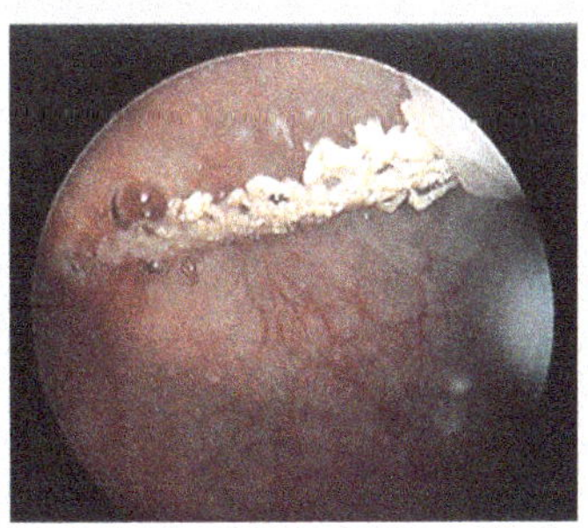

Figure 15.1 Cystoscopy of mesh in the bladder

Cystoscopy identifies the presence of mesh in the bladder from a previous retropubic mid-urethral sling.

Many urologists utilize cystoscopy in their evaluation of male LUTS, especially those considering invasive therapy. In concordance to the guidelines, they utilize it to assess prostatic size, the presence of a middle lobe, and to rule out other pathology. Both prostate size and configuration can influence treatment recommendations and therapeutic outcomes. Urethral stricture disease is also identified.

In general, cystoscopy has limited value in the assessment of female SUI, but it can be helpful in evaluating the short fibrotic "stove-pipe" urethra sometimes present in ISD patients. The presence of such may influence treatment recommendations and outcomes.

Cystoscopic assessment of urethral length can be useful. A short urethra may complicate placement of a sub-urethral sling and is sometimes seen in prolapse patients and in those having had previous urethral surgery. Urethral length, angulation, and degree of descensus at rest may also make treatment with bulking agents more challenging.

Cystoscopy plays an important role in assessing patients with problems following bladder neck suspension. An upward urethral angle with an elevated "ski jump" effect at the bladder neck may suggest over correction from previous surgery. Mesh or foreign body in the bladder or urethra is easily identified.

Guidelines

We agree with the OAB guidelines that cystoscopy should not be used in the initial workup of the uncomplicated OAB patient.

Having said that, cystoscopy is beneficial in OAB patients who are refractory to medical therapy, and should also be performed in those reporting an acute change in lower urinary tract symptoms in the absence of other etiologies. Although rare, bladder cancer can present as a new onset of storage symptoms even in non-smokers and in the absence of hematuria.

Many patients with OAB report vague abdominal or pelvic discomfort. Others have more overt pain as part of their presentation, and may or may not have interstitial cystitis. In addition to ruling out other intravesical etiologies, duplication of the discomfort during cystoscopy may suggest the presence of bladder pain syndrome. Urethral tenderness and a low filling capacity may be suggestive of IC/BPS.

Cystoscopy plays an important role in evaluating many patients with voiding dysfunction. In fact, we view it as one of our voiding dysfunction stethoscopes.

In this population cystoscopy commonly identifies cloudy urine, white flecks and sediment, and diffuse bladder erythema, all in keeping with a chronic low grade bacterial cystitis that is likely been present for months or longer (Figure 15.2). From our experience, treatment followed by low dose antibiotic suppression will often eradicate the underlying cystitis and down-regulate the overactive bladder. Even those with severe symptoms can dramatically improve. For those who remain symptomatic, the usual OAB treatment pathway is recommended. It's important to control infections before you can successfully control urinary incontinence. Looking back, without cystoscopy, this patient type in many cases will go undiagnosed.

Figure 15.2 Cystoscopic view of cystitis and cloudy urine

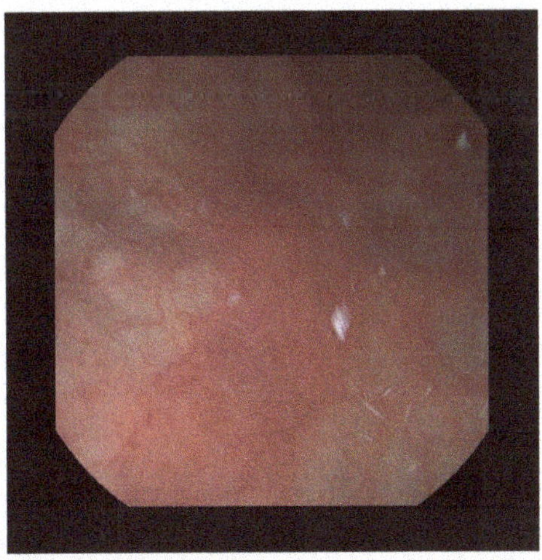

Cystoscopy should also be considered in female patients primarily reporting flow symptoms. Recognizing that it is not common, the presence of urethral stenosis can be identified. Carcinoma and other bladder or urethral pathology may present similarly.

Cystoscopy plays an important role in evaluating many patients with voiding dysfunction. In fact, we view it as one of our voiding dysfunction stethoscopes. Although normal findings are revealed in the majority, when pathology is identified, it's usually clinically relevant. But as is the case with urodynamics, often the only way to know if pathology exists is to do the evaluation.

Upper Tract Imaging

In general, upper tract imaging plays a minimal role in evaluating patients with voiding dysfunction. But, in select cases, it's important to image the upper tracts to rule out independent or related renal abnormalities.

We routinely recommend baseline renal ultrasound in many patients with neurogenic bladder dysfunction, especially those at risk of having poor bladder compliance and high filling or voiding pressures. Long-term surveillance with ultrasound performed annually or every two years is recommended.

The presence of silent hydronephrosis should be excluded in neurogenic patients, especially those with elevated post-void residuals. A firm PVR cut-off does not exist, but a more liberal approach is recommended versus the non-neurogenic population.

Importantly, women with severe vaginal vault prolapse may experience bilateral hydroureteronephrosis secondary to the prolapse. A renal ultrasound is adequate, but an unenhanced CT urogram may be more helpful in pre-operative planning, as it will detail ureteral anatomy and location (Figure 16.1–16.3). We don't routinely stent these patients, but are cognizant of the hydronephrosis during surgery.

> Importantly, women with severe vaginal vault prolapse may experience bilateral hydroureteronephrosis secondary to the prolapse. A renal ultrasound is adequate, but an unenhanced CT urogram may be more helpful in pre-operative planning as it will detail ureteral anatomy and location.

The intraoperative cystoscopic observation of bilateral ureteral efflux is adequate to ensure ureteral integrity.

Women with unilateral vague flank discomfort, with or without a renal stone history, should be radiographically evaluated prior to lower urinary tract and prolapse surgery. Trouble-shooting a postoperative ureteral abnormality is much easier when you have baseline information available.

Many patients with voiding dysfunction also have recurrent UTI's.

Figure 16.1 Pelvic examination in women with severe vaginal vault prolapse

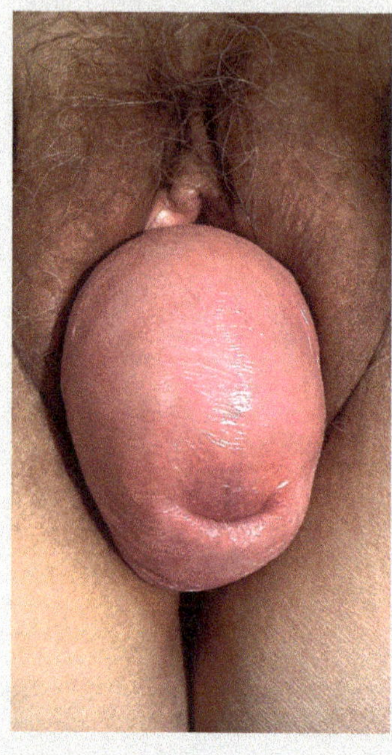

Figure 16.2 Renal ultrasound demonstrating bilateral hydronephrosis

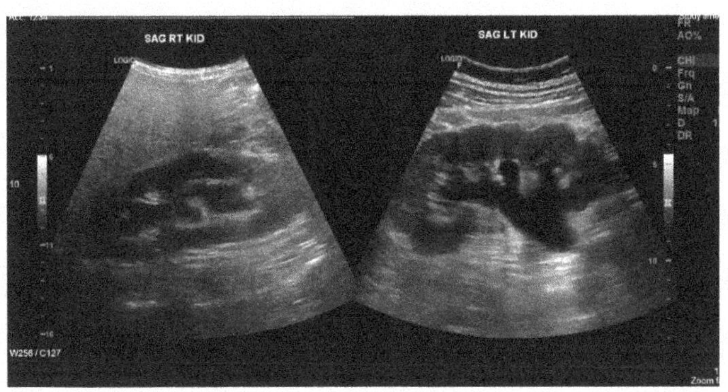

Figure 16.3 CT urogram diagnosing hydronephrotic ureters

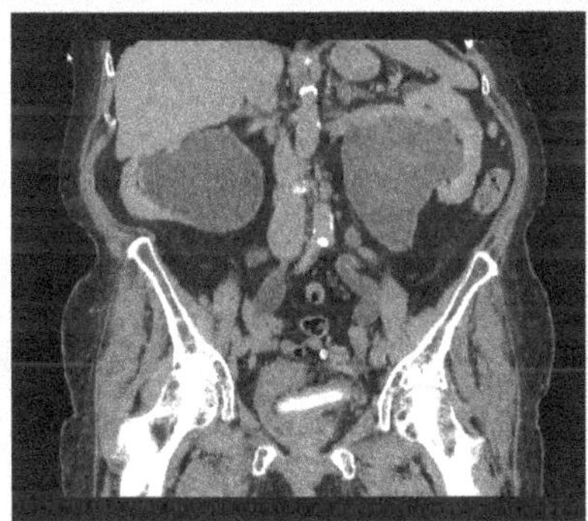

Guidelines

The UTI guidelines recommend that upper tract imaging should not be routinely obtained in the index patient presenting with a recurrent UTI.

We take a bullish approach in performing renal imaging in UTI patients, especially in those considering surgery for voiding dysfunction or prolapse. The use of imaging in more complicated UTI patients has been clearly established, but is beyond the scope of this discussion.

Overactive Bladder Syndrome (OAB): Diagnosis to Treatment Pathway

Many of the OAB patients we treat have complicating factors or underlying etiologies. They don't fit the pure OAB diagnosis but they present with the same symptoms. It's the presence of these "other factors" that may lead to a different diagnosis to treatment pathway in individual patients.

OAB diagnosis

The AUA OAB guidelines provide a clinical framework for the diagnosis of non-neurogenic overactive bladder. The following are the guideline statements regarding diagnosis.

Guidelines

The clinician should engage in a diagnostic process to document symptoms and signs that characterize OAB and exclude other disorders that could be the cause of the patient's symptoms; the minimum requirements for this process are a careful history, physical exam, and urinalysis.

In some patients, additional procedures and measures may be necessary to validate an OAB diagnosis, exclude other disorders and fully inform the treatment plan. At the clinician's discretion, a urine culture and/or post-void residual assessment may be performed and information from bladder diaries and/or symptom questionnaires may be obtained.

Urodynamics, cystoscopy and diagnostic renal and bladder ultrasound should not be used in the initial workup of the uncomplicated patient.

We value the guidelines but caution against their conservative presentation. We have already vetted the basic evaluation of patients with voiding dysfunction, and recommend the liberal use of urine cultures, post-void residuals, bladder diaries, and other diagnostic stethoscopes in patients with OAB.

Most OAB patients don't require urodynamics or cystoscopy but those with complicated, mixed, or less clear presentations should be evaluated. Risk factors, symptom severity, response to conservative treatment, and patient expectations should also be considered.

In a referral practice we commonly perform urodynamics and cystoscopy in OAB patients. As is the case with stress incontinence, it's the additional diagnostic findings that may redefine the patient's complexity retrospectively.

Urodynamics confirms the underlying bladder storage disorder and sheds light on its severity. It can identify an undiagnosed incompetent urethral sphincter or voiding disorder that may or may not be clinically relevant. The diagnosis of other underlying etiologies including painful bladder syndrome, neurogenic bladder dysfunction, and a small contracted bladder may also be suggested. These findings in turn influence the eventual diagnosis to treatment pathway.

OAB treatment

The AUA guidelines provide a framework for the treatment of OAB. Guideline statements concerning first, second, third, and fourth-line therapies are clearly presented. We would like to make a few additional comments, as well as discuss the OAB treatment pathway.

First-line therapies

Guidelines

Clinicians should offer behavioral therapies (e.g., bladder training, bladder control strategies, pelvic floor muscle training, fluid management) as first line therapy to all patients with OAB and that they may be combined with pharmacologic management.

We are advocates for behavioral therapy, but believe it is underutilized in clinical practice. It's noteworthy that the "first-line" therapy of a guideline statement is used minimally by many providers. Behavioral therapy is effective, but the treatment is time consuming and patient compliance varies.

Most clinicians prescribe an OAB agent as their primary treatment option. We offer medication with behavioral therapy to many of our patients first-line.

Second-line therapies

Guidelines

Clinicians should offer oral antimuscarinics or oral β3-adrenoceptor agonists as second-line therapy. If a patient experiences inadequate symptom control and/or unacceptable adverse drug events with one antimuscarinic medication, then a dose modification or a different antimuscarinic medication or a β3-adrenoceptor agonist may be tried.

Clinicians may consider combination therapy with an antimuscarinic and β3-adrenorecptor agonist for patients refractory to monotherapy with either antimuscarinics or β3-adrenoceptor agonist.

The majority of OAB patients are managed with medication. We prefer a β3-adrenoceptor agonist over an antimuscarinic because of its efficacy and tolerability. It's also safe in the elderly and frail. The FDA approval of a second B3-agonist has further strengthened our therapeutic armamentarium.

Antimuscarinics remain an excellent option, and a number of agents exist. Dose-escalation improves efficacy and is usually well tolerated in those having minimal side effects with the lower dose. There is increasing concern that antimuscarinics may be associated with memory loss and dementia, but more information is needed. The potential association of antimuscarinics with central nervous system side effects should be discussed with patients.

The patient response to OAB agents is heterogeneous. Their efficacy and tolerability varies greatly amongst individuals. Switching from one antimuscarinic to another or to a β3-agonist may improve efficacy or reduce side effects. The number of "switches" before declaring a patient as being refractory isn't clear, but we commonly try up to three agents. In patients who don't want medication or have contraindications, we advance to third-line treatments sooner.

The literature supports the efficacy and tolerability of combining a β3-agonist and antimuscarinic for the treatment of OAB. It's an excellent option for those who may or may not be considering third-line treatments. Less commonly, we combine two antimuscarinics in select patients.

Third-line therapies

Many OAB patients do not reach their treatment goal with behavioral therapy and medication. Refractory OAB or "ROAB" is arguably more common than OAB that is effectively managed by conservative approaches.

Guidelines

The AUA guideline panel defines the refractory patient as one who has failed a trial of symptom-appropriate behavioral therapy of sufficient length to evaluate potential efficacy and who has failed a trial of at least one antimuscarinic medication administered for 4 to 8 weeks.

In the patient who has failed behavioral and pharmacologic therapies or who is not a candidate for these therapies, onabotulinumtoxinA therapy, PTNS, or neuromodulation may be offered.

Clinicians may offer intradetrusor onabotulinumtoxinA (100U) as third-line treatment in the carefully-selected and thoroughly-counseled patient who has been refractory to first- and second-line OAB treatments. The patient must be able and willing to return for frequent post-void residual evaluation and able and willing to perform self-catheterization is necessary.

Clinicians may offer peripheral tibial nerve stimulation (PTNS) as third line treatment in a carefully selected patient population.

Clinicians may offer sacral neuromodulation (SNM) as third line treatment in a carefully selected patient population characterized by severe refractory OAB symptoms or patients who are not candidates for second-line therapy and are willing to undergo a surgical procedure.

We agree with the panel's refractory definition, but usually try more than one medication before recommending third-line therapies. Four weeks of treatment is generally long enough to assess efficacy and a lengthier trial only delays therapy.

We offer most patients the choice between onabotulinumtoxinA, PTNS, and SNM. We question the guideline's phraseology of patients having to be "carefully selected" since most can tolerate these reasonably non-invasive procedures. In the absence of a pacemaker or pregnancy, PTNS can be offered to nearly all patients. Patient selection for onabotulinumtoxinA and sacral neuromodulation requires more attention.

The eCoin tibial nerve stimulator was recently FDA approved for refractory overactive bladder, and we now offer it as a third-line therapy. Its efficacy and safety was clearly established in its pivotal study and we believe that it will soon be added to the AUA OAB guidelines. Because of its infancy in clinical practice, reference to it is limited in the modules, but the majority of comments made regarding sacral neuromodulation and PTNS also apply to it.

Many patients responding to third-line therapies still have residual symptoms and often benefit from reintroducing previously prescribed and partially effective oral agents. Likely one-third of our third-line patients are treated with this combination approach.

Fourth-line therapies

A number of patients fail first, second, and third-line OAB therapies. Many have severe symptoms, medical co-morbidities, or functional disorders associated. Augmentation cystoplasty and urinary diversion are available, but are less commonly performed in this population.

The OAB pathway

The OAB pathway or treatment algorithm has been popularized by urologists, especially those in large urology group practices. The pathway guides the patient through first, second, and third-line therapies, improving patient adherence and delivering excellent care. Guideline-based, each practice tailors the pathway depending on their treatment philosophy.

Maintaining and advancing patients through the pathway is important for success. Without a pathway, the utilization of third-line therapies is lower and fewer patients receive effective treatment. The penetrance of third-line therapies for the treatment of OAB in most practices is less than five percent.

Appropriate expectations and having patients aware of the pathway is paramount. Regular follow-up, quantitating response to therapy, and encouraging patients goes a long way in ensuring effective outcomes and high patient satisfaction.

In this OAB diagnosis to treatment module we will speak to the OAB pathway and how it's used and modified in individual female patients. The cases will highlight the usefulness of urodynamics and other testing in this population. The diagnosis and treatment of male OAB will be featured elsewhere.

CASE 1

Severe Refractory OAB

Diagnosis

History

Marilyn is a 81-year-old woman with a four year history of urgency incontinence. She denies stress incontinence and enuresis but reports 'leaking all the time.' Even with repeat questioning, characterizing her incontinence and voiding dysfunction is difficult.

She wears eight to 10 pads daily that are moderately wet or soaked. She double pads when she is out in public, and has limited her activity.

The patient voids every one to two hours and has no nocturia. She experienced minimal benefit from a β3-agonist and has failed two antimuscarinics.

Marilyn has a number of medical comorbidities and ambulates well with a walker. She reports mild vague lower abdominal pressure unchanged with urination. She denies a history of UTI's and has not had previous bladder surgery. Her incontinence is significantly impacting her quality of life.

Marilyn has refractory OAB and is bothered by her severe symptoms. Especially in the elderly, we routinely perform cystoscopy in refractory patients looking for the presence of occult cystitis and other less common intravesical etiologies. We don't perform urodynamics in all ROAB patients but are very liberal in doing so. Refractory OAB can be difficult to treat, and a better understanding of the patient's voiding dysfunction can be helpful in recommending the best diagnosis to treatment pathway.

Based on Marilyn's refractory and severe symptoms, urodynamics were recommended. With her history being less clear, the study's objectiveness may also play an important role in her assessment.

Physical exam

On pelvic examination, the patient has mild urethral and bladder neck hypermobility but no demonstrated SUI with a weak cough. She has mild vaginal atrophy and no prolapse. She is moderately overweight and ambulates well with a walker.

Post-void residual urine volume

3 mL

Urinalysis

Rare bacteria, few WBC's, 0 RBC's

Cystoscopy

Marilyn (A)

During cystoscopy the patient had impressive diffuse bladder erythema associated with cloudy urine and white flecks. The urothelial changes were in keeping with cystitis and not carcinoma in situ. As a result, the urine was sent for culture and urodynamics were postponed.

Marilyn (B)

Normal cystoscopic findings. In the absence of an intravesical etiology, the patient was evaluated with urodynamics.

Urodynamics

Marilyn (B)

During urodynamics, the patient had a MCC of 464 mL associated with mild increased bladder sensation. She had one involuntary detrusor contraction reaching a pressure of 9 cmH$_2$O associated with mild urgency incontinence. Her cough leak point pressure was 12 cmH$_2$O at 100 mL, and she leaked a moderate amount. Pressure flow and electromyography was within normal limits (Figure M1-1).

Figure M1-1: Marilyn (B) urodynamics

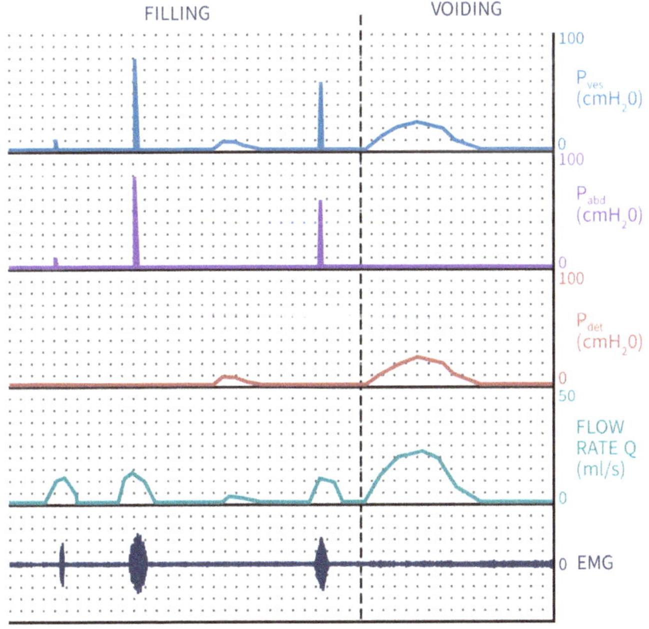

Diagnosis

Marilyn (A and B) have severe refractory UUI and urinary frequency. They have failed two prior antimuscarinics and partially responded to a β3-agonist. Characterizing their incontinence during the history was challenging.

Marilyn (A)

Cystoscopy identified occult cystitis in the absence of symptoms or past history of UTI's. A positive urine culture confirmed the diagnosis. Having a positive culture associated with a normal urinalysis has been well described.

Marilyn (B)

Patient was evaluated with urodynamics. She has normal bladder capacity and mild increased bladder sensation. She has low pressure detrusor overactivity associated with mild incontinence and favorable bladder storage characteristics. She has significant ISD even at low bladder volumes. Based on the study her 'leaking all the time' is likely due to urethral incompetence versus an overactive detrusor.

The literature supports that up to 34% of women with a negative clinical history of SUI subsequently are found to have stress incontinence. The detection of "occult stress incontinence" during urodynamics or physical exam is especially common in older patients. Even with subsequent questioning, Marilyn B continued to deny SUI.

Diagnosis to treatment pathway

The diagnosis to treatment pathway of Marilyn (A) and (B) are different based on their evaluation.

Marilyn (A)

- Marilyn (A) will be treated for a low grade UTI with the assumption that she's likely had it for months or longer. The undetected diagnosis may help explain why her OAB symptoms were refractory to previously tried medications.
- Following urine sterilization, Marilyn (A) will be placed on daily antibiotic prophylaxis and reassessed in 6–8 weeks. The UTI guidelines don't recommend a renal ultrasound, but we usually get one in this situation.

In a significant number of patients, their OAB improves on suppressive therapy. The down-regulation of even severe symptoms, including nocturia and enuresis, can be very substantial. Marilyn's vague abdominal pressure may cease if its referred discomfort from her low grade cystitis.

Although some patient's continence status immediately responds to the initial UTI treatment, most take several weeks on prophylaxis before realizing the benefit. This delayed response further supports the chronic nature of the underlying bladder infection.

The duration of prophylaxis remains unknown. Discontinuing within 6–12 months is reasonable knowing if symptoms return it may be due to recurrent infection. Others are kept on prophylaxis long-term.

If Marilyn (A) remains symptomatic on antibiotics she will reenter the OAB diagnosis to treatment pathway. Having failed previous medication, it's reasonable to consider combination therapy. Her initial partial response to a B3-agonist may improve with the urine sterilized especially when combined with an antimuscarinic. Otherwise, urodynamics will be ordered to help guide the next step.

Marilyn (B)

- The diagnosis to treatment pathway for Marilyn (B) is interesting. Without urodynamics, she would be offered third-line therapies likely favoring PTNS based on her age and comorbidities. OnabotulinumtoxinA and sacral neuromodulation are options and their consideration should be individualized. Without knowing that she has associated ISD, these refractory therapies would likely be less effective, and the patient may be disappointed with their outcome.
- Based on urodynamics, her diagnosis to treatment pathway changed. She has significant urethral insufficiency in combination with an overactive bladder. We would initially offer her a urethral bulking agent over a third-line therapy in an attempt to effectively manage her mixed presentation.

  For those who would treat Marilyn (B) with a third-line therapy, the patient should be aware that the efficacy of them is lower than what is to be expected in the index OAB patient due to the presence of her ISD.

Treating refractory OAB by addressing occult urethral incompetence is not new. Before the advent of effective third-line therapies, we commonly used bulking agents in this population with reasonable success. In the absence of the patient reporting SUI, justifying an invasive sling is difficult, but could be considered especially if bulking agents were temporarily successful.

Treating ISD may secondarily improve overactive bladder based on what is referred to as urethral relaxation incontinence. The ICS defines it as urethral relaxation in the absence of raised abdominal pressure or detrusor overactivity.[11] Once coined urethral instability, it's thought that urine entering the proximal incompetent urethra may secondarily trigger a detrusor contraction with incontinence. Its effective management with a bulking agent or bladder neck suspension may prevent the urethral reflex activity and associated leakage.

CASE 2

Urinary Incontinence Not Associated with Awareness

Diagnosis

History

Susan is a 54-year-old women who leaks a small amount with coughing and sneezing, but not with bending, lifting, and with other activities. She denies urgency incontinence but can leak without awareness while standing and sitting. She has no enuresis and wears three pads daily that are moderately wet or soaked.

The patient voids every one to two hours and has no nocturia. Her flow is sometimes good and other times poor. She often does not feel empty after urination.

She has no other complicating urologic factors, has minimal medical comorbidities, and has not been treated for her voiding dysfunction.

Susan reports stress incontinence and leakage not associated with awareness. The latter is often due to an overactive detrusor and is therefore included in this OAB module. Based on her presentation, urodynamics were performed. Four studies will be presented, as well as their recommended diagnosis to treatment pathway.

Physical exam

On pelvic examination, Susan has moderate urethral and bladder neck hypermobility but no demonstrated SUI. She has an asymptomatic small cystocele but no evidence of a urethral diverticulum.

Post-void residual urine volume

7 mL

Urinalysis

Normal

Urodynamics

Susan (A)

During urodynamics, the patient had a MCC of 542 mL with normal bladder sensation. She had no detrusor overactivity and demonstrated moderately severe urodynamic SUI at 220 mL with a LPP of 21 cmH$_2$O. Pressure flow and electromyography was within normal limits.

Susan (B)

During urodynamics, the patient had a MCC of 462 mL with normal bladder sensation (Figure M1-2). Cystometry demonstrated multiple detrusor contractions reaching a pressure of 7 cmH$_2$O that were not perceived by the patient. During one of the contractions she leaked her entire bladder volume, necessitating bladder refilling. She had urodynamic SUI leaking a few drops with a LPP of 151 cmH$_2$O only occurring near bladder capacity. Pressure flow and electromyography were within normal limits.

Figure M1-2: Susan (B) urodynamics

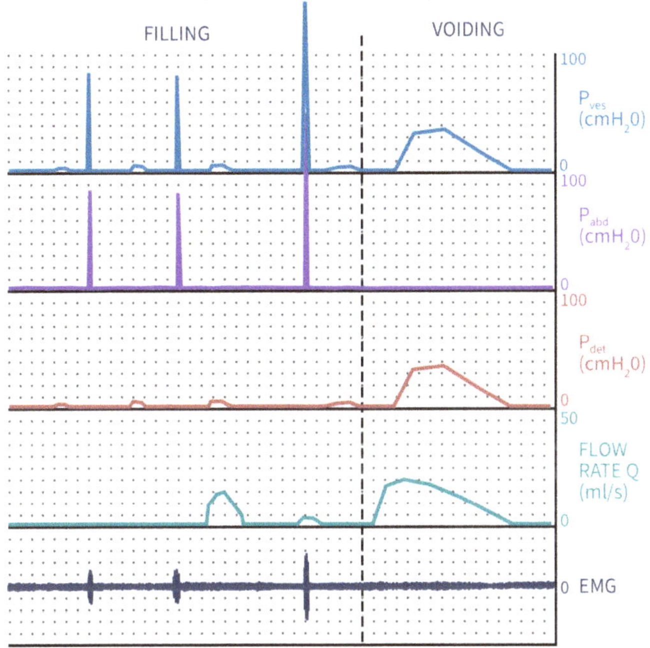

Susan (C)

During urodynamics, the patient had a MCC of 141 mL and increased bladder sensation. Cystometry demonstrated multiple detrusor contractions reaching a pressure of 27 cmH$_2$O associated with mild urgency. She was able to inhibit the majority and only leaked a few drops. She had urodynamic SUI leaking a small amount with a LPP of 137 cmH$_2$O. Pressure flow and electromyography were within normal limits.

Case 2 / Urinary incontinence not associated with awareness

Susan (D)

During urodynamics the patient had a MCC of 312 mL and increased bladder sensation. Cystometry demonstrated multiple detrusor contractions reaching a pressure of 16 cmH$_2$O associated with significant urgency incontinence. She had urodynamic SUI with a LPP of 40 cmH$_2$O leaking a moderate amount. Pressure flow and electromyography were within normal limits.

Diagnosis

Susan (A–D) report stress urinary incontinence and leakage without awareness. They do not have overflow incontinence or evidence of a urethral diverticulum.

Susan (A)

During urodynamics, Susan (A) has normal bladder filling and a low leak point pressure leaking a moderate amount at low bladder volumes.

Her ISD explains her stress incontinence and leakage not associated with awareness. In the absence of other causes, we are confident that Susan (A)'s urethral incompetence is the underlying problem.

Susan (B)

Based on the urodynamics, Susan (B) has a different diagnosis. Her filling cystometry clearly demonstrates that detrusor overactivity is the cause of her insensate urine loss. Her high LPP explains her mild stress incontinence, but not her leakage while standing and sitting.

On further questioning, Susan (B) reports other symptoms supporting an overactive bladder. Sometimes when she turns on a tap, urine runs down her leg and she can soak a pad while quietly sitting. It's these high volume episodes that are most bothersome to her.

Susan (C)

Susan (C) has unfavorable bladder storage characteristics on filling cystometry. She has a markedly reduced bladder capacity and significant detrusor overactivity. She has mild urodynamic SUI and high abdominal leak point pressures.

It's likely that Susan (C)'s insensate leakage is from an overactive detrusor and not from her mild SUI. Although the study didn't reproduce the symptom it appears to be the diagnosis by exclusion.

Susan (D)

Susan (D) has significant detrusor overactivity and ISD, and we believe that either one could cause her incontinence not associated with awareness. Both her overactive detrusor and urethral incompetence are contributing to her clinical presentation.

Diagnosis to treatment pathway

Susan (A–D) report mild stress incontinence and insensate urine loss while standing and sitting. Based on urodynamics their diagnosis to treatment pathway differ.

Susan (A)

- Susan (A) will be offered the recommended non-surgical and surgical treatment options for the index SUI patient. Based on her favorable bladder storage characteristics and normal voiding, she appears to be an excellent surgical candidate.

Susan (B)

- Susan (B) primarily has an overactive detrusor and will be managed with the OAB pathway. Her mild SUI will be treated with pelvic floor muscle training.
- If Susan (B) fails medical and behavioral therapy, she will be offered third-line OAB treatments and not a sling. If her mild SUI is ever managed surgically, she is at risk of having persistent postoperative incontinence not associated with awareness.

Susan (C)

- Based on urodynamics, the diagnosis of Susan (B) and (C) are similar. Susan (C)'s leakage without awareness is from an overactive detrusor and not her mild SUI. Her diagnosis to treatment pathway would mirror that of the previous patient.

Susan (D)

The diagnosis to treatment pathway of Susan (D) is challenging. She has moderately severe SUI, and her insensate urine loss may be due to either an overactive detrusor or an incompetent sphincter.

- Susan (D) will be offered medical and behavioral therapy directed towards her "mixed" picture. If she fails, both third-line OAB therapies and SUI treatments will be discussed.
- If Susan (D) consents to a sling or bulking agent, she will realize that her insensate urine loss may persist, especially if it's secondary to detrusor overactivity. If she chooses a refractory OAB treatment, it will not address her stress incontinence. Neither path clearly addresses both symptoms, and having appropriate patient expectations is important.

CASE 3

OAB-Dry

Diagnosis

History

Keila is a 41-year-old women with urinary frequency worsening over 12 months. She voids every 30 to 45 minutes, and can't sit through a two-hour movie without urinating. She is continent and gets up twice during the night to void.

She urinates frequently because of bladder fullness. She has intermittent suprapubic pressure that's relieved by voiding, but denies pelvic pain and dyspareunia. She has a reduced flow and a feeling of incomplete emptying.

Prior to this, Keila was voiding four or five times daily. She can't identify a precipitating cause of her change in voiding function.

Her bowel function is normal, and she has had a previous hysterectomy. She is otherwise healthy and has not been treated for her voiding dysfunction.

Keila has impressive urinary frequency and mild nocturia, which represents a significant change in her voiding function. Her presentation is somewhat out of the ordinary, hence both cystoscopy and urodynamics were recommended. Three studies will be presented as well as their recommended diagnosis to treatment pathway.

Physical exam

On pelvic examination, Keila has a well-supported urethra and bladder neck and no demonstrated SUI. She has no bladder and pelvic floor muscle tenderness.

Post-void residual urine volume

16 mL

Urinalysis

Normal

Cystoscopy

During cystoscopy, the bladder mucosa and trigone were normal. She had no evidence of carcinoma, occult cystitis, or foreign body related to her hysterectomy. She felt immediate fullness during bladder filling but did not experience pelvic pain.

Urodynamics

Keila (A)

During urodynamics the patient had a MCC of 160 mL limited by bladder fullness and pressure. She was uncomfortable and could not tolerate further bladder filling. She had no detrusor overactivity or urodynamic SUI. Pressure flow and electromyography were within normal limits.

Keila (B)

During urodynamics the patient had a MCC of 322 mL and increased bladder sensation. She had decreased bladder compliance with an end filling pressure of 21 cm H_2O. She had repetitive detrusor overactivity reaching a pressure of 47 cmH$_2$O and leaked a small amount. She had no urodynamic SUI generating abdominal pressures of 130 cmH$_2$O. During voiding her P$_{det}$max was 38 cmH$_2$O and the Qmax was 11 mL/sec. EMG activity increased and her flow pattern was prolonged.

Keila (C)

During urodynamics the patient had a MCC of 387 mL with mild increase in bladder sensation. She had detrusor overactivity reaching a pressure of 14 cmH$_2$O but did not leak. She had no urodynamic SUI generating abdominal pressures of 138 cmH$_2$O. During voiding her P$_{det}$max was 27 cmH$_2$O and the Qmax was 10 mL/sec. EMG activity increased during voiding, and her flow pattern was intermittent and prolonged.

Diagnosis

Keila (A–C) have significant urinary frequency with mild nocturia and normal cystoscopy.

Keila (A)

Keila (A) has significantly reduced bladder capacity limited by bladder fullness and suprapubic pressure. Although she doesn't report pain, her unfavorable filling cystometry supports the possibility of her having interstitial cystitis.

The AUA IC/BPS guidelines recommend hydrodistension as third-line therapy, but we routinely use it diagnostically. It's especially useful in patients like Keila (A) who have an atypical presentation. The cystoscopic findings supporting an IC diagnosis can be impressive, even in those with milder or nonspecific symptoms.

Keila (A)'s hydrodistension demonstrated severe and diffuse glomerulations associated with mild mucosal bleeding (Figure M1-3). Her bladder capacity under anesthesia was 440 mL and she had no Hunner's ulcers. Subsequently, she was diagnosed with having interstitial cystitis.

Figure M1-3:
Photo of IC Bladder

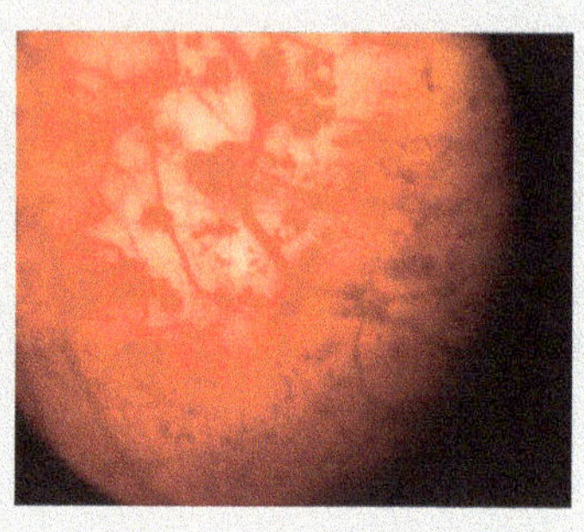

Keila (B)

Keila (B) has high pressure detrusor overactivity and decreased bladder compliance, suggesting the possibility of her having a neurogenic bladder. Her high voiding pressure, reduced flow rate, and external sphincter dyssynergia also support the diagnosis.

Keila (B) was referred to neurology for further evaluation. Keila was subsequently diagnosed as having a congenital spinal cord abnormality that is followed conservatively.

Keila (C)

During urodynamics Keila (C) has normal bladder capacity and an overactive detrusor. She has favorable bladder storage characteristics and no urodynamic SUI. Her voiding pressure is normal, but she has a prolonged reduced flow secondary to external sphincter dyssynergia.

Keila (C)'s urodynamics support the diagnosis of OAB-dry. Her pelvic floor dyssynergia explains her reduced flow and may be contributing to her overactive bladder.

Diagnosis to treatment pathway

Based on urodynamics and subsequent evaluation, each individual Keila has a different diagnosis to treatment pathway.

Keila (A)

Keila (A) has interstitial cystitis with urinary frequency and a feeling of incomplete bladder emptying. Without pelvic pain, her presentation is somewhat atypical.

- Keila (A) will be offered the various treatment options recommended by the AUA IC/BPS guidelines. With symptomatic management being the primary goal, OAB medications and sacral neuromodulation are important treatment options.

The driving symptom of OAB is urgency. In contrast, those with an inflamed bladder typically report pain or "pressure" which may or may not be relieved by voiding. The differentiation between fullness, urgency, pressure, and pain can be subtle, but the underlying etiology and its management is vastly different. We believe that "painless IC" does exist and should be suspect in patients with severe frequency and a feeling of incomplete bladder emptying.

Keila (B)

- Keila (B) has a neurogenic bladder and will be managed using the OAB pathway. In spite of her unfavorable bladder storage characteristics, she can still respond to OAB medications. Rarely, these agents cause reduced flow or urinary retention in the neurogenic population. Third-line therapies are effective in managing OAB symptoms in patients with neurogenic lower urinary tract dysfunction.

- Keila (B)'s high filling and voiding pressure places her at higher risk of upper tract deterioration. A renal ultrasound is recommended and should be repeated long-term.

Keila (C)

Keila (C)'s urodynamics support the diagnosis of OAB-dry. Idiopathic overactive bladder is the most common diagnosis but does not apply to all.

- Keila (C) will be treated with the OAB pathway. Bladder retraining will be emphasized to reeducate her reduced functional bladder capacity. Pelvic floor muscle therapy directed towards her pelvic floor dyssynergia may improve her flow as well as her OAB symptoms.
- OAB agents are the primary treatment of OAB-dry. Sometimes they can be discontinued after several months of successful bladder retraining. Third-line therapies are effective, but some may be considered too invasive in this scenario. Percutaneous tibial nerve stimulation is a good option to consider in those with milder symptoms.

CASE 4

Detrusor Hyperactivity with Impaired Contractility (DHIC)

Diagnosis

History

Martha is a 77-year-old women with urgency incontinence. She voids every one to two hours and gets up once during the night to urinate. She denies both stress incontinence and enuresis. She wears four wet pads per day to manage her incontinence. Her flow is reasonable, and she feels empty after urination.

When her bowel movements are loose, she may experience mild fecal incontinence not associated with awareness. She reports vaginal pressure and is not sexually active.

She has a history of recurrent UTI's and is otherwise healthy. She has not been treated for her voiding dysfunction.

Martha has moderately severe urgency incontinence. She has intermittent fecal incontinence and reports mild prolapse symptoms. Because her post-void residual was elevated during her initial evaluation, both cystoscopy and urodynamics were subsequently recommended. Three studies will be presented as well as their recommended diagnosis to treatment pathway.

Physical exam

On pelvic examination the patient has mild urethral and bladder neck hypermobility and no demonstrated SUI. She has significant vaginal atrophy and no prolapse. Her anal sphincter tone is normal and she has no evidence of fecal impaction.

Post-void residual urine volume

261 mL

Urinalysis

Normal

Cystoscopy

During cystoscopy the bladder mucosa and trigone were normal. She had no intravesical abnormalities or evidence of urethral or meatal stenosis.

Urodynamics

Martha (A)

During urodynamics, the patient had a MCC of 660 mL and normal bladder sensation. She had detrusor overactivity reaching a pressure of 12 cmH_2O and associated with mild urgency incontinence. She had no urodynamic SUI. During voiding, she generated a poorly sustained detrusor contraction reaching a P_{det}max of 7 cmH_2O. She voided 400 mL with a Qmax of 6 mL/sec and her PVR was 283 mL. The EMG activity was normal (Figure M1-4).

Figure M1-4: Martha (A) urodynamics

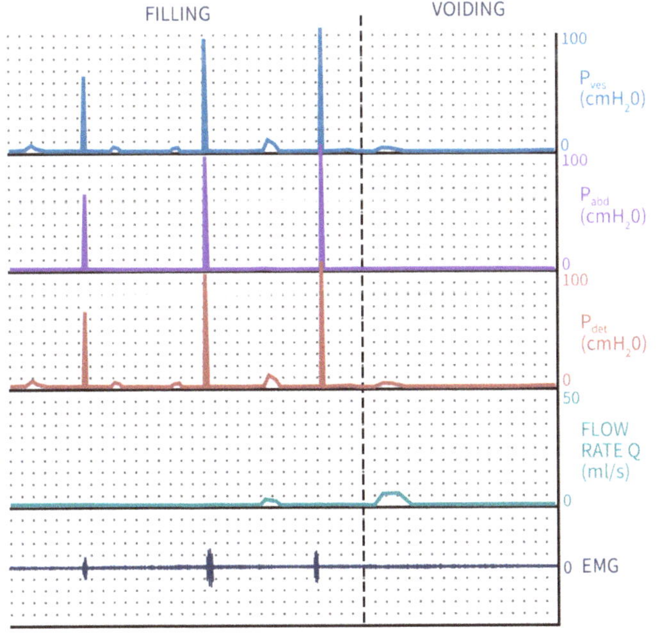

Martha (B)

During urodynamics, the patient had a MCC of 387 mL limited by urgency incontinence. She had repetitive detrusor overactivity reaching a pressure of 14 cmH$_2$O and associated with high volume leakage. She had no urodynamic SUI. During voiding the P$_{det}$max was 52 cmH$_2$O and the Qmax was 4 mL/sec. She voided 190 mL and her PVR was greater than 200 mL. EMG activity increased during voiding and her flow pattern was prolonged (Figure M1-5).

Figure M1-5: Martha (B) urodynamics

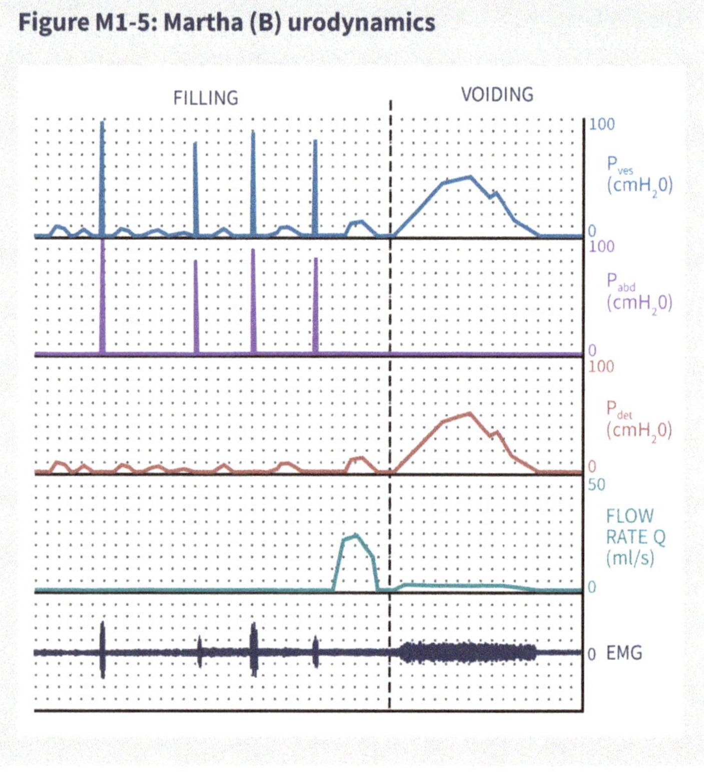

Martha (C)

During urodynamics the patient had a MCC of 917 mL and decreased bladder sensation. She had detrusor overactivity reaching a pressure of 4 cmH_2O associated with mild leakage. She demonstrated urodynamic SUI with a LPP of 134 cmH_2O leaking a few drops at volumes greater than 600 mL. During voiding, she could not generate a detrusor contraction and voided by abdominal straining. Her Qmax was 18 mL/sec and the PVR was 212 mL. The EMG activity increased, and her flow pattern was intermittent and prolonged.

Diagnosis

Martha (A–C) have urgency incontinence associated with an elevated post-void residual. They have an overactive bladder as well as fecal incontinence.

Based on physical examination and cystoscopy, Martha (A–C) have no anatomic cause of their incomplete bladder emptying. In the absence of pelvic organ prolapse, their vaginal pressure is likely secondary to atrophy. Local estrogen replacement therapy can be successful in ameliorating these symptoms.

Urgency incontinence associated with elevated residuals is especially common in the elderly. Originally called detrusor hyperreflexia with impaired contractility (DHIC), the ICS has since described the condition as the concurrence of detrusor overactivity (DO) with detrusor underactivity (DU).[12] As described, the impaired emptying is due to diminished detrusor contractile function and is associated with bladder trabeculation, a slow velocity of bladder contraction, little detrusor reserve power, and a significant amount of residual urine. Many providers use the term DHIC loosely to describe patients with urgency incontinence and elevated residuals, regardless of the underlying bladder dysfunction.

Case 4 / Detrusor hyperactivity with impaired contractility (DHIC)

Martha (A)

Martha (A) fits the original DHIC definition. She has urgency incontinence secondary to an overactive detrusor and an elevated residual due to impaired bladder contractility. The incomplete emptying exacerbates the OAB symptoms, especially in those with reduced functional capacities. A renal ultrasound is important to consider to rule out the presence of hydronephrosis.

Martha (B)

Martha (B) has detrusor overactivity and urgency incontinence. She is urodynamically obstructed and has excellent detrusor reserve power. In the absence of a neurologic diagnosis or anatomic obstruction, her elevated residual is due to external sphincter and pelvic floor dyssynergia.

Martha (C)

Martha (C) has a different underlying bladder dysfunction or arguably a more severe "DHIC" presentation. She has low pressure detrusor overactivity with urgency incontinence. She has a large capacity acontractile bladder and strains to urinate. Her intermittent increased EMG activity is due to abdominal straining and not from pelvic floor dyssynergia. Her urodynamic SUI is mild and is likely not clinically relevant.

Diagnosis to treatment pathway

Martha (A–C) have urgency incontinence with incomplete bladder emptying. Based on urodynamics, their diagnosis to treatment pathway is different.

We initially focus the treatment of Martha (A–C) at improving bladder emptying.
A combination of behavioral therapy and α-adrenergic receptor antagonists is recommended.

- Behavioral techniques including double voiding, positional changes, and gentle Credé maneuvers can be successful in select patients. Bending forward combined with Credé voiding may especially benefit Martha (C) who has a large capacity acontractile bladder.

- Pelvic floor muscle relaxation to assist voiding should be recommended to Martha (B) who has pelvic floor dyssynergia. Having said that, it may tip the balance and improve bladder emptying in all patients with elevated PVR's.

- Bladder retraining and urgency suppression can increase functional bladder capacity and improve OAB symptoms in spite of high residuals. Some patients report improved flow and emptying when they void at higher volumes.

- Dietary modifications and behavioral therapy are proven strategies for fecal incontinence, but this discussion is beyond the scope of this diagnosis to treatment module.

- Although the concentration of alpha receptors in the female bladder neck and urethra is lower than men, women may still respond favorably to α-adrenergic receptor antagonists. We routinely prescribe alpha blockers to females with flow symptoms, with or without elevated residuals, and find them beneficial in a significant minority. Symptoms often improve even though their PVR may remain unchanged.

When alpha blockade fails, Martha (A–C) are then managed by the OAB pathway.

- The elevated residual is accepted, and they are symptomatically managed with OAB agents. A β3-agonist is preferred since its associated risk of causing urinary retention appears lower than with antimuscarinics.

- We still use antimuscarinics in this population, and don't hesitate to dose-escalate or use in combination with β3-agonists. Urinary retention is surprisingly rare, but patients should be followed long-term for increasing residuals. Some patients with loose bowel movements and fecal incontinence respond favorably to antimuscarinics.

The treatment pathway of Martha (A–C) may vary when it comes to recommending third-line OAB therapies.

- *Sacral neuromodulation (SNM)* is FDA approved for both urgency and fecal incontinence. In small studies it has been shown to be effective in DHIC patients like Martha (A), demonstrating satisfactory success in treating both the detrusor hyperactivity and impaired contractility components of the condition.

  Although it's known that SNM addresses pelvic floor dysfunction, it's not been studied in a large cohort of patients like Martha (B) who has an elevated PVR. Similarly, its effectiveness in Martha (C), who has a large capacity acontractile bladder, has not been established. SNM appears to be a good treatment option for both patients, recognizing that its success rate may be less than an index patient. OAB symptoms can improve with or without a change in the post-void residual urine volume.

- *Percutaneous tibial nerve stimulation* can be effective in managing Martha (A–C)'s urgency incontinence, but its effects on bladder emptying is unknown. It's approved in Europe for fecal incontinence, but not in the U.S.

   We have extensive experience with PTNS and routinely use it in OAB patients with elevated residuals. Many are elderly with medical comorbidities and respond well to the office-based procedure. PTNS manages the symptoms, but usually does not improve the PVR.

- OnabotulinumtoxinA is a treatment option for patients with OAB, but should be used with caution in Martha (A–C), who have elevated residuals. In the pivotal trials, the retention rate was 6.5% in idiopathic OAB patients who had a baseline PVR of less than 100 mL.

   In small DHIC studies, onabotulinumtoxinA did not increase the rate of urinary retention but appeared to be less effective. The baseline PVR in these studies was only modestly elevated, and the results should not be generalized to the entire DHIC population.

   Many experts don't recommend onabotulinumtoxinA in patients whose PVR is greater than 250 mL, unless they are willing to accept the high risk of retention and perform clean intermittent catheterization. Based on their underlying bladder dysfunction, knowing which Martha (A–C) is at highest risk of retention with onabotulinumtoxinA remains unknown.

Female Stress Urinary Incontinence (SUI): Diagnosis to Treatment Pathway

Many female patients with stress urinary incontinence (SUI) have complex presentations, while others are more simple, some of them being referred to as an index patient.

Guidelines

The AUA stress urinary incontinence guidelines define the index patient as an otherwise healthy female who is considering surgical therapy for the correction of pure stress and/or stress-predominant mixed urinary incontinence and who has not undergone previous surgery. Patients with low-grade pelvic organ prolapse are also considered to be index patients.

The guidelines recommend that in the initial evaluation of index patients with SUI desiring to undergo surgical intervention, physicians should include the following components:

- *History, including assessment of bother*
- *Physical examination, including a pelvic examination*
- *Objective demonstration of SUI with a comfortably full bladder (any method)*
- *Assessment of post-void residual urine (any method)*
- *Urinalysis*

We agree with the guidelines but caution that many patients in clinical practice who meet the index definition are actually more complicated.

It takes just a few additional symptoms or findings to potentially increase complexity, and these complicating factors may be subtle.

We are concerned that the index recommendations may be generalized and applied to more complicated patients and bias care beyond the guideline's specified narrative. Many patients benefit from urodynamics, which can alter their diagnosis to treatment pathway. It's the urodynamic findings that in many cases redefine the complexity of the patient retrospectively.

This diagnosis to treatment module will concentrate on a number of SUI patients we commonly see in clinical practice. Our hope is to provide you with a real world experience that demonstrates the benefit of urodynamics in this population.

CASE 1

Index SUI Patient

Diagnosis

History

Sally is a 61-year-old woman who presents with urinary incontinence. Her primary complaint is leaking during coughing, sneezing, golfing, and when lifting her grandchildren.

She voids every three hours and infrequently gets up once a night to urinate. She wears 3 pads daily that are usually damp, but sometimes moderately wet when golfing.

Sally has no other complicating urologic factors, has minimal comorbidities, and has not been treated for her voiding dysfunction.

Sally has stress urinary incontinence worse when she is active. We will discuss her as an index patient and share with you some thoughts regarding workup and treatment.

We agree with the guidelines that Sally's basic evaluation should include a history, physical, urinalysis, and measurement of the post-void residual urine volume. Preoperative urodynamics is optional, but is routinely performed by many. Doing a functional test for a functional problem before functional surgery is a reasonable doctrine to follow.

We perform urodynamics in nearly all of our surgical SUI patients. Even subtle abnormalities may change the diagnosis to treatment pathway. Urodynamic findings can be valuable and alter the surgical consent discussion. Preoperative urodynamics can also make troubleshooting any postoperative problems easier.

Physical exam

On pelvic examination Sally has moderate urethral and bladder neck hypermobility leaking a small amount. She has no prolapse, and her vagina is reasonably well estrogenized. She is mildly overweight and has no cognitive or functional problems.

Post-void residual urine volume

22 mL

Urinalysis

Normal

Diagnosis

Sally has a diagnosis of stress urinary incontinence and meets the definition of an index patient.

Diagnosis to treatment pathway

Guidelines

We agree with the SUI guidelines that patients wishing to undergo treatment of SUI, that the degree of bother that their symptoms are causing them should be considered in their decision for therapy. The patient has a number of treatment options available.

- *Observation*
- *Pelvic floor muscle training (+/− biofeedback)*
- *Other non-surgical options (continence pessaries and vaginal inserts are recommended by the AUA)*
- *Surgical intervention*

Pelvic floor muscle training (PFMT)

Pelvic floor muscle training (PFMT) can be highly effective. We provide in-office physical therapy and it has been an excellent addition to our practice. The majority of patients we refer respond favorably and don't advance to more invasive treatments.

Non-surgical options

Urologists have less experience with non-surgical devices for the treatment of SUI, and they may be more popular in gynecology practices. Options include continence pessaries and vaginal inserts. The use of pessaries is generally limited to pelvic organ prolapse.

Guidelines

In index patients considering SUI surgery, physicians may offer the following options:
- *Mid-urethral synthetic sling*
- *Autologous fascia pubovaginal sling*
- *Burch colposuspension*
- *Bulking agents*

Mid-urethral synthetic slings

The surgical gold standard for SUI is the synthetic mid-urethral sling. In spite of issues involving mesh, it is an effective and durable procedure. In experienced hands, the complications are minimal and arguably easier to manage versus those occurring with other bladder neck suspensions.

The retropubic or transobturator sling are the literature-based options for the index patient. The single-incision sling is an alternative, but the patient should be made aware that its long-term efficacy has not been established.

Autologous fascia pubovaginal sling

The guidelines recommend using autologous fascia over cadaveric fascia and porcine dermis based on efficacy. We don't think that the literature supporting a superiority claim is strong enough to justify the added morbidity of the fascial harvest and commonly use cadaveric fascia.

Burch colposuspension

We have a lot of experience with the Burch colposuspension and are aware of its benefits and risks. In spite of its proven value, it's difficult to justify to patients who are not already undergoing an abdominal procedure. A laparoscopic procedure can be considered based on the surgeon's experience.

Bulking agents

Bulking agents are a recommended treatment for SUI, even in those with urethral hypermobility. They are easy to perform, office-based, and are an excellent option for those wishing to avoid surgery or having concerns regarding the longer postoperative recovery. Commonly used as a salvage procedure, their utilization first-line has been limited by their lower efficacy and high retreatment rates. Newer bulking agents are available, and the treatment paradigm appears to be changing. Many providers are now offering them as a good first line alternative, although the long-term data in the U.S. is still pending.

There is a popular viewpoint that all surgical options should be offered to SUI patients. Although this is reasonable, we caution that patients may not be able to make the best decision, since the issue is so complex. Strongly biased by "I don't want mesh," the patient unknowingly may choose a more morbid procedure, or one that has its own inherent problems.

In contrast, we recommend to offer the procedure that, in the surgeon's hands, is best for the individual patient. We would recommend Sally a mid-urethral sling and a urethral bulking agent as a less invasive alternative. We recommend the pubovaginal sling in select cases and have not performed a Burch colposuspension in years.

If Sally was managed with pelvic floor muscle training, we generally schedule a 4-month follow-up to monitor her progress. It's important to evaluate whether or not she has reached her treatment goal with non-surgical therapy.

CASE 2

Index Patient with Urinary Frequency

Diagnosis

History

Jane is a 64-year-old woman who presents with urinary incontinence. Her primary complaint is leaking during coughing, sneezing, getting out of a chair, and especially with laughing. She has an urgent bladder but no urgency incontinence.

She voids every one to two hours, and gets up twice during the night to urinate. She wears 3 pads daily that are usually damp but sometimes soaked.

Jane has no other complicating urologic factors, has minimal comorbidities, and has not been treated for her voiding dysfunction.

Jane meets the definition of an index patient. She has SUI with urinary frequency and nocturia but no obvious complicating factors. In addition to the basic workup, she was evaluated with urodynamics. Urodynamics will be included as part of the workup in the next several cases.

Physical exam

On pelvic examination, the patient has moderate urethral and bladder neck hypermobility leaking a small amount. She has no prolapse, and her vagina is reasonably well estrogenized. She is mildly overweight and has no cognitive or functional problems.

Post-void residual urine volume

16 mL

Urinalysis

Normal

Urodynamics

Jane (A)

During urodynamics, the patient had a MCC of 514 mL associated with normal bladder sensation. She had mild urgency during filling but no involuntary detrusor overactivity. Her cough leak point pressure was 70 cmH$_2$O at 200 mL associated with moderate urodynamic SUI. Pressure flow and electromyography were within normal limits.

Jane (B)

During urodynamics the patient had a MCC of 220 mL limited by fullness and urgency. She had multiple overactive detrusor contractions reaching a pressure of 22 cmH$_2$O associated with significant urgency incontinence. Her cough leak point pressure was 162 cmH$_2$O leaking a few drops at 200 mL. Pressure flow and electromyography were normal (Figure M2-1).

Figure M2-1: Jane (B) urodynamics

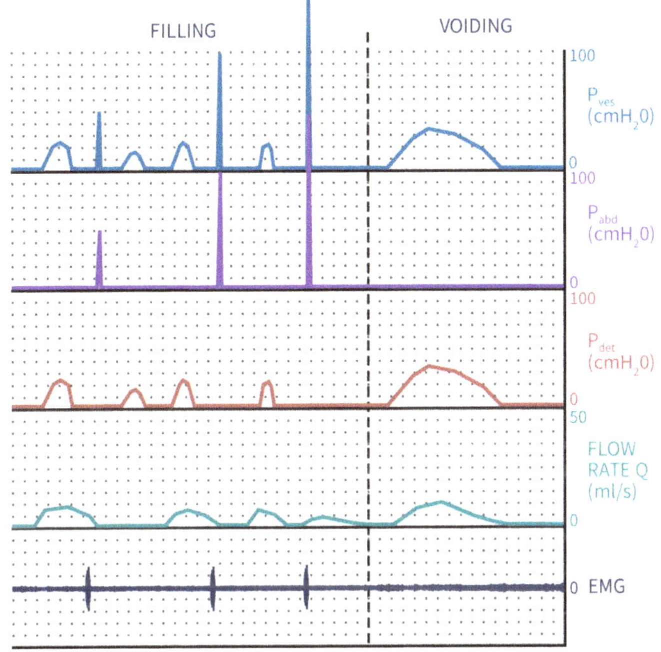

Diagnosis

Jane (A) and (B) have a diagnosis of stress urinary incontinence and meet the definition of an index patient. They have urinary urgency and frequency or OAB-dry as well as nocturia.

Jane (A)

Jane (A)'s urodynamics demonstrate SUI and normal bladder filling and emptying. The findings correlate with her presentation and support the clinical diagnosis. At this stage, the surgeon can be confident walking Jane (A) through their usual narrative when consenting her for a bladder neck suspension.

Jane (B)

Jane (B) presented with a diagnosis of SUI with urgency and frequency, but has a markedly abnormal filling cytometry. The urodynamics don't correlate well with her presumed diagnosis and instead shine the light on her bladder storage disorder.

It's important to dissect each symptom and how it correlates with the urodynamic findings. By doing so, it appears that Jane (B) has a clinically significant overactive bladder and mixed urinary incontinence.

Her leaking with coughing and sneezing is from bladder neck hypermobility and SUI. But based on her high LPP's and leaking only a few drops, her incontinence getting out of chair and while laughing is probably due to triggered bladder overactivity and not from urethral incompetence.

Considering that Jane (B)'s urodynamic SUI is mild, her "soaked" episodes are likely secondary to detrusor overactivity and not stress incontinence. With further questioning, if she reports urine "running down her leg" when she goes from a sitting to standing position or incontinence persisting even after she stops laughing, you likely have confirmed her OAB diagnosis.

Jane (B)'s frequency and nocturia are similarly due to an overactive bladder. Her frequent voiding may be protecting her from otherwise experiencing urgency incontinence at higher bladder volumes.

Diagnosis to treatment pathway

The diagnosis to treatment pathway is different for Jane (A) and (B).

Jane (A)

- Jane (A) will be offered the recommended non-surgical and surgical options for the index patient with SUI.

Jane (B)

- The treatment of Jane (B) will be directed towards her mixed symptoms. She will be started on behavioral therapy, pelvic floor muscle training, and OAB medications.
- If Jane (B) doesn't reach her treatment goal with medical and behavioral therapy, then surgical management of her mixed symptoms will be recommended. She has clinically significant SUI, and we would offer her a sling or bulking agent over a third-line OAB therapy for her mixed presentation.

During the consent process, she will be cautioned that any symptom attributable to OAB could persist or worsen following an incontinence procedure. For example, Jane (B)'s frequency, giggle incontinence, and high volume episodes triggered by getting out of a chair could persist postoperatively. In addition to her having realistic expectations, knowledge of her overactive bladder will make trouble-shooting easier if she remains symptomatic postoperatively. A detailed approach in how we consent the mixed SUI/UUI patient considering bladder outlet surgery will be presented in the mixed incontinence diagnosis to treatment module.

Without performing urodynamics in this index patient there, would be no individual Jane (A) and Jane (B). Both Janes would appear the same and likely be treated with with a stress incontinence procedure. Jane (A) probably would have responded to surgical correction. Jane (B)'s pathophysiology may not have been addressed properly, and her OAB may have persisted . Persistent or worsening symptoms attributable to an overactive bladder following a sling can result in a dissatisfied patient as well as a physician who now has stress.

CASE 3

Index Patient with Flow Symptoms

Diagnosis

History

Andrea is a 53-year-old woman who presents with urinary incontinence. Her primary complaint is leaking during coughing, sneezing, and exercising. She has no urgency incontinence.

She voids every three to four hours and has no nocturia. She wears three pads daily that are moderately wet. Her flow is sometimes poor and other times reasonable. She double voids a small amount and usually feels empty.

Andrea has no other complicating urologic factors, has minimal comorbidities, and has not been treated for her voiding dysfunction.

Andrea meets the definition of an index patient. Her flow symptoms are non-specific and common. She does not appear to have significant voiding dysfunction that would recategorize her as being non-index according to the guidelines. In spite of this, she did have urodynamics as part of her diagnostic evaluation.

Physical exam

On pelvic examination the patient has moderate urethral and bladder neck hypermobility leaking a small amount. She has no prolapse and her vagina is reasonably well estrogenized. She is mildly overweight and has no cognitive or functional problems.

Post-void residual urine volume

72 mL

Urinalysis

Normal

Urodynamics

Andrea (A)

During urodynamics, the patient had a MCC of 580 mL associated with normal bladder sensation. She had mild urgency during filling but no involuntary detrusor overactivity (Figure M2-2).

Figure M2-2: Andrea (A) urodynamics

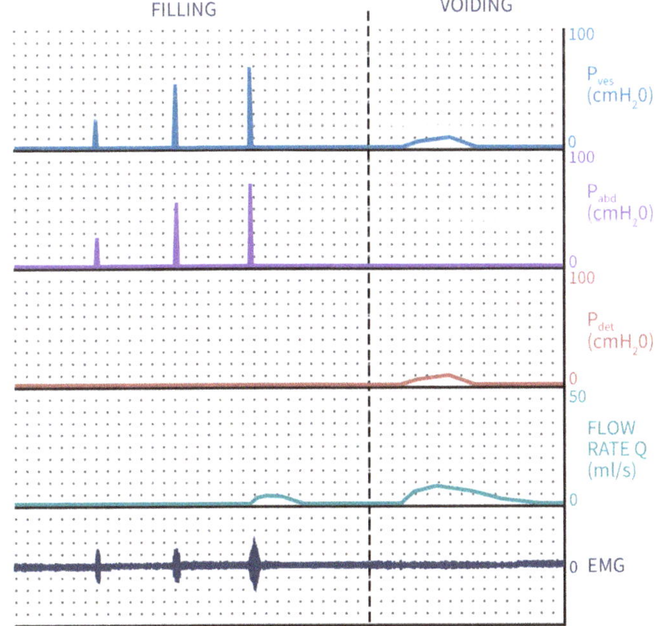

Her cough leak point pressure was 70 cmH$_2$O at 400 mL associated with moderate urodynamic SUI. During pressure flow her P$_{det}$max was 12 cmH$_2$O and the Qmax was 18 mL/sec. The flow pattern was mildly depressed but reasonably normal. Electromyography activity remained stable during voiding and the PVR was 23 mL.

Andrea (B)

During urodynamics, the patient had a MCC of 950 mL limited by bladder volume. During filling, she had significantly decreased bladder sensation and only reported mild fullness. No detrusor overactivity was demonstrated. Her cough leak point pressure was 70 cmH$_2$O at 400 and 650 mL with both associated with moderate leakage. During voluntary voiding, she did not demonstrate a detrusor contraction and voided by abdominal straining. Her Qmax was 18 mL/sec and her PVR was 23 mL. The flow pattern was spiking and intermittent, and her EMG activity increased during straining.

Diagnosis

Andrea (A) and (B) have a diagnosis of stress urinary incontinence and meet the definition of an index patient. They have mild to moderate nonspecific flow symptoms, and their initial postvoid residual is within normal limits.

Andrea (A)

Andrea (A)'s urodynamics demonstrate normal bladder filling and urodynamic SUI. Her voiding pressure and flow rate are mildly depressed but common in women with or without flow symptoms.

Many "normal" female voiders like Andrea (A) don't generate strong detrusor contractions during voiding, but empty efficiently be relaxing their pelvic floor. In addition, the EMG activity when measured by patch electrodes commonly remains stable during voiding in normal patients. In the absence of significant obstructive symptoms or other complicating factors (neurogenic bladder, elevated PVR, etc.), these findings don't increase the risk of developing urinary retention following a bladder neck procedure.

Andrea (B)

Andrea (B) has stress urinary incontinence but an abnormal filling cystometry and pressure flow evaluation. She has a large capacity bladder with markedly decreased bladder sensation. In spite of multiple attempts, she was not able to generate a voluntary detrusor contraction.

Upon further questioning, Andrea (B) describes her voiding pattern as straining. She commonly uses a Crede maneuver and gently bends forward in order to empty. She may not be able to void well without straining.

Diagnosis to treatment pathway

Both Andrea (A) and (B) have stress urinary incontinence but their diagnosis to treatment pathway is different based on their urodynamics.

Andrea (A)

- Andrea (A) will be offered the recommended non-surgical and surgical options for the index SUI patient. Although she has nonspecific flow symptoms and mild urodynamic findings, we would offer her a sling or bulking agent without any reservation. In the absence of other symptoms or abnormalities, we don't believe that she is at increased risk of postoperative urinary retention.

Andrea (B)

In contrast, the treatment of Andrea (B) is influenced by her abnormal filling and voiding study. Recognizing the absence of supporting data, she is at greater risk of developing retention following a bladder neck suspension.

- Andrea (B) will be encouraged to consider pelvic floor muscle training or a urethral bulking agent versus a sling. The risk of permanent retention with bulking agents approaches zero even in those with poor voiding characteristics.
- If Andrea (B) is treated surgically, some would argue for a transobturator approach over a potentially more obstructive V-shaped retropubic mid-urethral or pubovaginal sling. When tensioning the mesh during surgery, setting the sling a little bit looser is reasonable to consider to prevent poor emptying.

The urodynamics identified two different individuals versus one Andrea index patient. Although Andrea (B)'s true risk of retention is unknown, it is certainly greater than the 1–2% risk commonly quoted for slings. She is also at higher risk of developing worsening postoperative flow symptoms even if she can empty.

Bothersome flow symptoms, postoperative urinary retention, the need for prolonged clean intermittent catheterization, and a subsequent urethrolysis are significant concerns for both patient and surgeon. Any factor that could help predict or prevent this risk is clinically important. The only way to identify Andrea (B) from Andrea (A) is to do urodynamics prior to surgery in index patients.

Index Patient with Moderate to Severe SUI

Diagnosis

History

Samantha is a 56-year-old woman who presents with urinary incontinence. Her primary complaint is leaking during coughing, bending, walking, and activity. She has no urgency incontinence.

She voids every two to three hours and has no nocturia. She wears 6–8 pads daily that are moderately wet and sometimes soaked. Her urinary flow is reasonable and she feels empty after voiding.

Samantha has a history of recurrent UTI's and lumbar disc disease. She has had two lower back surgeries to address the problem.

She has no other complicating urologic factors, has minimal comorbidities, and has not been treated for her voiding dysfunction.

Samantha has stress urinary incontinence especially when she is active. Importantly, she had high volume urinary incontinence and even leaks with walking. Even though she has a history of recurrent UTI's and previous lumbar surgery, she still meets the definition of being an index patient.

Physical exam

On pelvic examination, the patient has minimal urethral and bladder neck hypermobility leaking a large amount. She has no prolapse and her vagina is reasonably well estrogenized. She is mildly overweight and has no cognitive or functional problems.

Post-void residual urine volume

14 mL

Urinalysis

Normal

Urodynamics

Samantha (A)

During urodynamics the patient had a MCC of 485 mL associated with normal bladder sensation. She had mild urgency during filling but no involuntary detrusor overactivity. Her cough leak point pressure was 62 cmH$_2$O at 400 mL associated with mild to moderate urodynamic SUI. Pressure flow and electromyography were within normal limits.

Samantha (B)

During urodynamics, the patient had a MCC of 485 mL associated with normal bladder sensation. She had mild urgency during filling but no involuntary detrusor overactivity. Her cough leak point pressure was 11 cmH$_2$O at 200 and 400 mL associated with high volume urodynamic SUI. Pressure flow and electromyography were within normal limits.

Samantha (C)

During urodynamics, the patient had a MCC of 485 mL associated with normal bladder sensation. She demonstrated multiple involuntary detrusor contractions reaching pressures of 18 cmH$_2$O consistently triggered by coughing and Valsalva. Each contraction was associated with moderate urinary incontinence. Otherwise, she had no SUI generating abdominal pressures of 120 cmH$_2$O. Pressure flow and electromyography was within normal limits (Figure M2-3).

Figure M2-3: Samantha (C) urodynamics

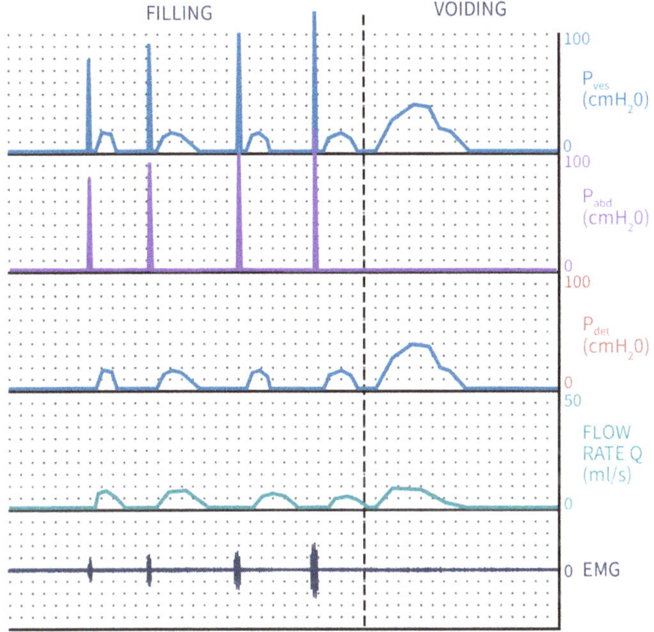

Samantha (D)

During urodynamics the patient had a MCC of 140 mL limited by suprapubic pain during bladder filling. She had no involuntary detrusor overactivity and was very uncomfortable during the study. Her cough leak point pressure was 92 cmH$_2$O at 100 mL leaking a small amount. During pressure flow her P$_{det}$max was 26 cmH$_2$O and the Qmax was 10 mL/sec. The EMG activity significantly increased during voiding, and her flow pattern was prolonged and intermittent. Her abdominal pain was relieved by voiding, but she had urethral soreness secondary to the catheter.

Samantha (E)
During urodynamics the patient had a MCC of 485 mL associated with normal bladder sensation. Her bladder compliance was decreased with an end filling pressure of 18 cmH_2O at bladder capacity. During filling she had a few low pressure involuntary detrusor contractions reaching a pressure of 6 cmH_2O felt as mild urgency. Her cough leak point pressure was 92 cmH_2O at 400 mL with moderate leakage. During pressure flow her P_{det}max was 48 cmH_2O and the Qmax was 8 mL/sec. EMG activity increased during voiding, and she had a prolonged flow pattern.

Diagnosis

Samantha (A-E) have a diagnosis of stress urinary incontinence, and meet the definition of an index patient. They have high volume leakage and a distant history of recurrent UTI's and lumbar disc surgery.

Samantha (A)
Samantha (A)'s urodynamics demonstrate normal bladder filling and emptying and a leak point pressure in keeping with her presentation. The urodynamic findings support her index status.

Samantha (B)
Samantha (B) similarly has urodynamic SUI and normal bladder filling and emptying. She has a low leak point pressure and leaks a large amount even at low bladder volumes.

Upon further questioning, not only does Samantha (B) leak during walking and activity she's incontinent sitting and rolling over in bed. She states that she "leaks all the time" and double pads during strenuous exercise in order to manage her incontinence.

Samantha (C)
Samantha (C) did not demonstrate urodynamic SUI generating abdominal pressures of 120 cmH_2O. Instead, she had impressive

detrusor overactivity triggered by coughing and Valsalva associated with moderate volume leakage.

Samantha (C) admits that when she leaks with coughing that urine will continue to run down her leg even after she stops coughing. She sometimes experiences urgency during these episodes.

Samantha (D)

Samantha (D) demonstrated urodynamic SUI but has markedly reduced bladder capacity and significant pain during filling. During voiding she has reduced flow secondary to pelvic floor dyssynergia. Her urodynamics and tender urethra support the diagnosis of painful bladder syndrome.

In retrospect, Samantha (D) experiences suprapubic pain associated with urinary frequency several times annually. Her symptomatic flares usually settle spontaneously while others are treated as a UTI with varying benefit. Urine cultures have not been sent by her primary physician to confirm the diagnosis. She has mild dyspareunia, especially during UTI episodes.

Samantha (E)

Samantha (E) has urodynamic SUI with abnormal bladder filling and voiding characteristics. She has decreased bladder compliance and low pressure detrusor overactivity. She is urodynamically obstructed secondary to external sphincter dyssynergia.

If fluoroscopy was performed, she might have a heavily trabeculated irregularly shaped bladder and bladder outlet obstruction at the level of the rhabdosphincter. The presence of spinal hardware may also be noted.

With further questioning, Samantha reports mild pins and needle sensation primarily in her lower extremities. She does not have vaginal or perineal numbness, and her bowel movements are reasonably normal.

Diagnosis to treatment pathway

Samantha (A-E) have stress urinary incontinence, but their diagnosis to treatment pathway are influenced by the urodynamic findings.

Samantha (A)

- Samantha (A) will be offered the recommended non-surgical and surgical options for the index SUI patient. Although she has a history of recurrent UTI's and previous back surgery, they are not complicating her index presentation.

Samantha (B)

Samantha (B) has intrinsic sphincter deficiency based on her clinical evaluation. She has an impressively low LPP and leaks a large amount even at low bladder volumes.

- *The authors agree with the SUI guidelines that the recommended treatment of ISD is a retropubic mid-urethral sling, a pubovaginal sling, or bulking agent.* Trans-obturator slings and a Burch colposuspension that address urethral hypermobility are associated with lower success rates in this population.

Many surgeons perform a transobturator or single-incision sling first-line in the majority of index patients. Without routine preoperative urodynamics and measurement of LPP it appears that they may not be offering the best procedure to patients like Samantha (B).

Samantha (C)

The diagnosis to treatment pathway for Samantha (C) should be reconsidered based on her urodynamics. Her history and physical support the diagnosis of SUI, but the urodynamic results bring this diagnosis into question. Although trigged DO is a common urodynamic finding, its clinical relevance is less clear. Having said that, it does challenge what is the best treatment strategy for the patient.

- We recommend for Samantha (C) to be initially treated with behavioral therapy, pelvic floor muscle training, and OAB medications. If she doesn't reach her treatment goal then SUI surgical options would be recommended. Discussion regarding the possibility of having persistent postoperative incontinence secondary to triggered detrusor overactivity should be emphasized.

Samantha (D)

The diagnosis to treatment pathway for Samantha (D) is clearly altered by her urodynamics. Her small capacity painful bladder and pelvic floor dyssynergia strongly support the diagnosis of chronic interstitial cystitis. Her reported UTI's were likely IC flares and, in retrospect, she has other symptoms suggestive of the diagnosis.

The literature supports that millions of women with IC are undiagnosed especially those with milder or nonspecific symptoms. The diagnosis may become apparent following a successful bladder neck suspension. The patient's postoperative ability to hold more urine can unmask their painful bladder, or the surgery itself may up-regulate pelvic pain pathways.

- The initial diagnosis to treatment pathway for Samantha (D) is directed towards her IC/BPS. A multimodal approach is recommended, including dietary measures and education, oral medications, bladder instillations, and pelvic floor physical therapy. Bladder hydrodistension is another treatment option, and we routinely use it to help make the diagnosis.

  When IC/BPS patients are effectively managed, they may report significant improvement in their voiding dysfunction, even stress urinary incontinence. We try to avoid surgery, because it could worsen their pain or voiding symptoms. Urethral bulking agents are an excellent treatment alternative in this population.

- If a bladder neck suspension is planned, it's best to do so when the painful bladder has been reasonably well-managed. Not only could surgery up-regulate pain, IC patients are likely at higher risk of retention due to their pelvic floor dyssynergia.

Samantha (E)

Samantha (E) appears to have a neurogenic bladder based on her urodynamic findings, having an impact on her diagnosis to treatment pathway.

- As a general rule, we caution against performing a sling in patients with neurogenic bladder dysfunction. Their detrusor overactivity will likely persist or worsen, and they are at higher risk of urinary retention.
- As a consequence, pelvic floor muscle training and bulking agents will be recommended to address Samantha (E)'s stress incontinence. And based on her poor bladder compliance, her upper tracts will be evaluated by a screening renal ultrasound and followed long-term.

By performing urodynamics prior to surgery, patients like Samantha (B–E) will be identified. Although some findings are more common than others, many patients turn out to be more complicated than how they initially appear. The history and physical exam, PVR, and urinalysis will not identify these patients, and the only way to diagnose them is to routinely perform urodynamics.

Female Mixed Urinary Incontinence: Diagnosis to Treatment Pathway

Approximately 50% of the women with stress incontinence will have OAB symptoms. The literature supports that the prevalence of mixed symptoms is high, and it significantly impacts quality of life. Most experts agree that mixed patients can be challenging to treat. The contribution of OAB dry or OAB wet to the symptom bother or to the urinary loss may vary, thus complicating the treatment pathways. Data regarding mixed incontinence management based on the heterogeneity of symptoms and urodynamics is limited, and hence the associated guideline statements are sparse.

Guidelines

Regarding diagnosis, physicians should perform additional evaluations in patients being considered for surgical intervention who have urgency-predominant mixed urinary incontinence. Physicians may also perform additional evaluations in SUI patients with concomitant overactive bladder symptoms.

Beyond the guidelines that primarily apply to the index SUI patient there are no guideline statements specifically addressing the maLEAVE THE SAMEnagement of mixed patients.

Patients with mixed stress and urgency incontinence are not all the same. There is a spectrum of patients ranging from those who primarily have stress incontinence and mild UUI to those with symptoms mainly attributable to an overactive bladder and who have mild SUI. In the

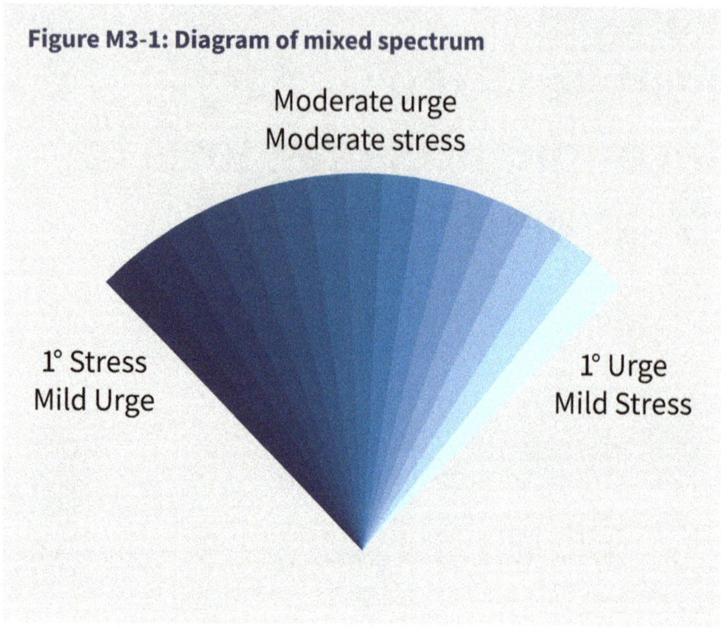

Figure M3-1: Diagram of mixed spectrum

middle of the spectrum are those who have a more 50:50 distribution (Figure M3-1). The symptom that is most bothersome creates additional variability when evaluating each individual.

Recognizing the spectrum, it's naive to think that all mixed patients would have the same diagnosis to treatment pathway and respond similarly to treatment. For example, a sling is an excellent option for women with mixed incontinence when the predominant cause is stress incontinence, but not for the patient with mild SUI and large volume urgency incontinence and flooding bedwetting.

Identifying where each individual presents on the spectrum is important. Quantifying the contribution of each type of incontinence includes the severity, the bother, and patient expectations from treatment. Because the bladder is an unreliable witness, we believe that a basic evaluation is insufficient, and we recommend a thorough history and physical examination combined with urodynamics to best define the mixed patient.

The objective urodynamics findings of how well the bladder stores, and how incompetent is the outlet are correlated with the patient's symptoms and physical exam. When the findings all align, the clinician is more confident of the etiology of the symptoms, signs, and objective urodynamic findings. When there is discordance, we recommend to re-evaluate and validate the findings, explain the discrepancy, and to proceed with caution.

In many of the patients with predominant stress incontinence and OAB-dry, the treatment pathway is straightforward. However, in the more complex presentation of symptoms, the history is not always the best representation of the patient's underlying pathophysiology. The physical exam contributes additional data. However, many times the urodynamic findings better define the voiding dysfunction. Using all of the data and employing a constantly-questioning and conservative approach provides a more informed basis for recommending an effective diagnosis to treatment pathway.

In the more complex patient, urodynamics is essential. The urodynamic evaluation needs to be focused and performed meticulously, especially in the patient with potential detrusor overactivity and severe ISD. It may be necessary to repeat the cystometry in an attempt to elicit detrusor overactivty. In the patient with an incompetent outlet, it is important to make sure they are not leaking around the urodynamic catheter during bladder filling and affecting pressure measurements.

In this module we will present a number of studies that will demonstrate the benefit of urodynamics in mixed patients. In each urodynamic study, we will concentrate primarily on how well the bladder stores and how incompetent is the outlet. For simplicity, the patient's ability to empty will be normal.

We will emphasize not only initial management but also treatment beyond conservative approaches. Urodynamics will help guide decision making along the various steps of the diagnosis to treatment pathway.

CASE 1

Patient with Moderate Stress and Urgency Incontinence

Diagnosis

History

Wendy is a 66-year-old woman who presents with mixed urinary incontinence. She leaks with coughing, sneezing, and during most activities. She has urgency incontinence and key-in-the-door syndrome. She wears 4 pads daily that are moderately wet, and both the stress and urgency components are significant and bothersome.

She voids every one to two hours and gets up once at night to urinate. Wendy has no other complicating urologic factors, has minimal comorbidities, and has not been treated for her voiding dysfunction.

Wendy has mixed stress and urgency incontinence. In addition to the basic workup, she was evaluated with urodynamics. A number of studies will be presented as well as their recommended diagnosis to treatment pathway.

Physical exam

On pelvic examination, the patient has moderate urethral and bladder neck hypermobility leaking a small amount. She has no prolapse, and her vagina is reasonably well estrogenized. She has no cognitive or functional problems.

Post-void residual urine volume

4 mL

Urinalysis

Normal

Urodynamics

Wendy (A)

During urodynamics, the patient had a MCC of 566 mL associated with normal bladder sensation. She had moderate urgency during filling, but no involuntary detrusor overactivity. Her cough leak point pressure was 24 cmH$_2$O at 300 mL associated with high volume urodynamic SUI. Pressure flow and electromyography were within normal limits (Figure M3-2).

Figure M3-2: Wendy (A) urodynamics

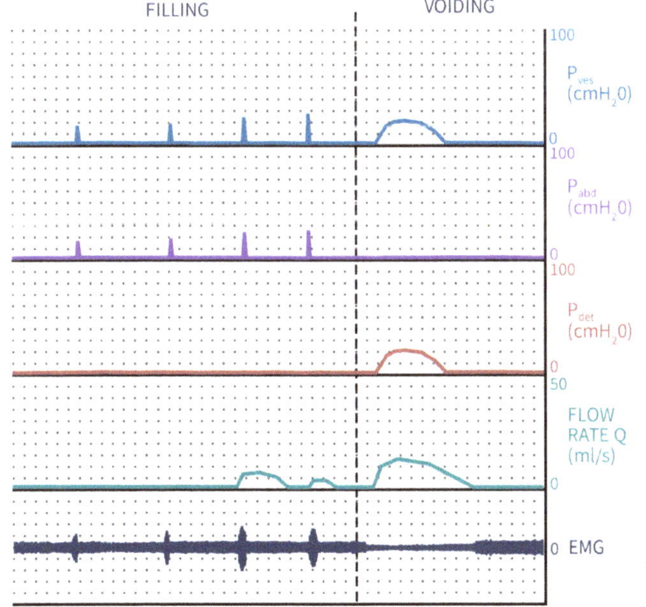

Wendy (B)

During urodynamics, the patient had a MCC of 144 mL associated with increased bladder sensation. She had impressive involuntary detrusor overactivity reaching pressures of 49 cmH$_2$O associated with high volume incontinence. She did not leak generating abdominal pressures of 112 cmH$_2$O with repetitive coughing. Pressure flow and electromyography were within normal limits (Figure M3-3).

Figure M3-3: Wendy (B) urodynamics

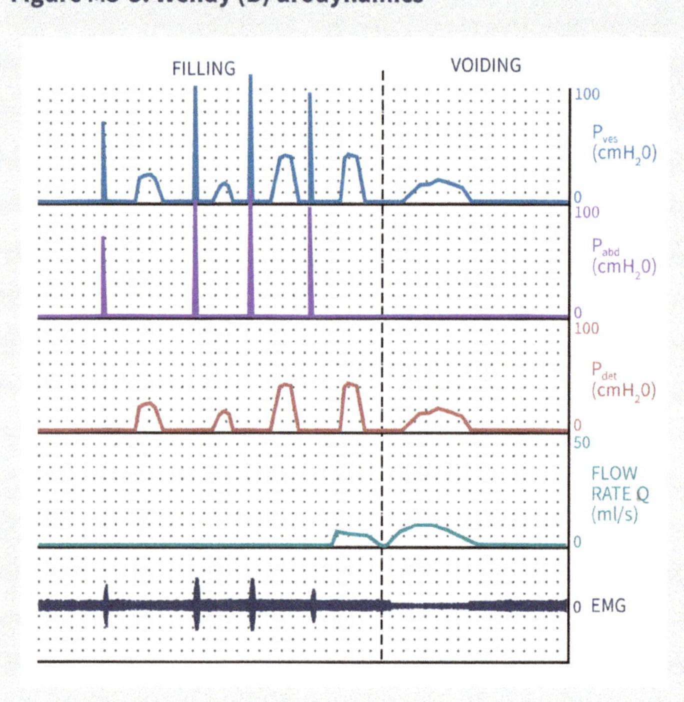

Wendy (C)

During urodynamics, the patient had a MCC of 463 mL and normal bladder sensation. She had moderate urgency incontinence due to involuntary detrusor overactivity reaching pressures of 28 cmH$_2$O. Her cough leak point pressure was 70 cmH$_2$O at 200 mL associated with moderate urodynamic SUI. Pressure flow and electromyography were within normal limits (Figure M3-4).

Figure M3-4: Wendy (C) urodynamics

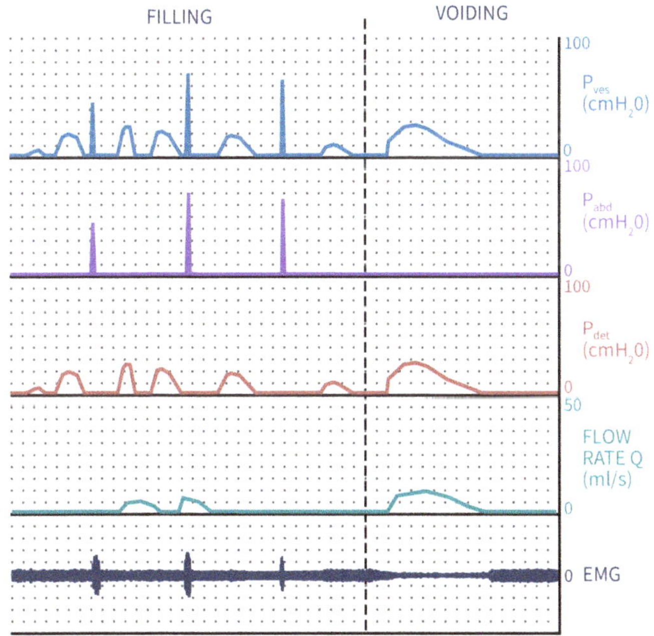

Wendy (D)

During urodynamics, the patient had a MCC of 164 mL and increased bladder sensation. She had repetitive involuntary detrusor overactivity reaching pressures of 22 cmH$_2$O. In most cases her DO was associated with urgency incontinence or leakage not associated with awareness. She had no urodynamic SUI generating abdominal pressures of 156 cmH$_2$O. Pressure flow and electromyography were within normal limits (Figure M3-5).

Figure M3-5: Wendy (D) urodynamics

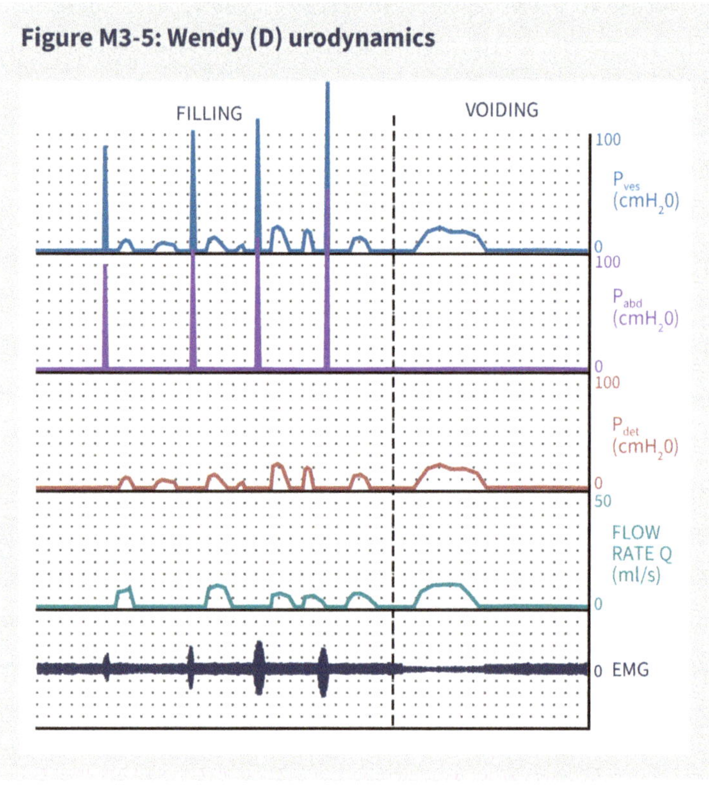

Diagnosis

Wendy has a diagnosis of mixed urinary incontinence. She has moderately severe leakage, and reports that both types of incontinence are significant and bothersome. She has mild urinary frequency and nocturia.

Wendy (A)

Wendy (A) has a normal filling cytometry and demonstrated moderately severe urodynamic SUI with a low leak point pressure. She has favorable bladder storage characteristics in combination with intrinsic sphincter deficiency.

Wendy (B)

Wendy (B) has a markedly reduced bladder capacity and impressive detrusor overactivity associated with significant incontinence. Based on her urodynamics her SUI is mild and it appears to occur at abdominal pressures greater than 112 cmH_2O. Many women with SUI cannot generate a high enough abdominal pressure during the study to elicit the symptom.

Wendy (C)

Wendy (C) demonstrates both moderately severe detrusor overactivity with incontinence, as well as moderate urodynamic SUI. The findings correlate well with the patient's initial presentation.

Wendy (D)

Wendy (D) has a small capacity bladder demonstrating significant detrusor overactivity, and leaking with urgency and without awareness. No urodynamic SUI could be demonstrated at an abdominal pressures of 156 cmH_2O.

Diagnosis to treatment pathway

Before discussing Wendy (A–D)'s individual diagnosis to treatment pathway, we would like to further discuss the female mixed patient.

First-line therapy

Prior to the advent of multiple newer OAB medications, many patients with mixed incontinence were treated with surgery first-line. The effectiveness of surgery for the OAB component was variable and, in many cases, the symptoms persisted and sometimes worsened. Now surgery is performed less often as first-line therapy.

We recommend OAB agents and behavioral therapy as first-line treatment in the majority of patients with mixed incontinence. OAB medications are the treatment of choice, especially in those with significant storage symptoms. Medication can also be effective in those with stress-predominant mixed symptoms. How many OAB agents to try is tailored to the individual.

In our experience most patients are eager to avoid surgery and appreciate conservative measures. This initial non-surgical approach highlights the presence of their OAB and its subsequent possible persistence in those who are eventually managed surgically. When symptoms persist postoperatively, troubleshooting is easier and patients are more understanding.

The refractory mixed patient

How to best manage "refractory mixed incontinence" deserves discussion. It's the patient with mixed symptoms who has not reached their treatment goal with medical and behavioral therapy. The question is whether to offer them surgery for stress incontinence or third-line OAB treatment as the next step.

We regularly perform stress incontinence surgery in refractory mixed patients. Based on experience and soft historical data, we use an "index mixed patient template" to counsel them regarding surgical outcomes.

The success rate of a sling for the SUI component approaches 90%. Approximately 10% of the successes are not completely SUI free, but the patients are satisfied with the outcome. Surgery for stress incontinence fails in approximately 10% of cases. The general consensus is that urgency incontinence improves in approximately two thirds of mixed patients treated with surgery for stress incontinence. OAB symptoms persist in one third and worsen in approximately 1–2%.

This outcome data is only a template on which to begin a discussion and should be tailored to the individual. For example, telling a patient that their flooding bedwetting or that their severe urgency incontinence secondary to a stroke will respond to a sling in 65% of cases is not in the patient's best interest. Clearly, the index numbers should be adjusted based on the patient's history, physical, urodynamics, and other clinical factors.

It's important for patients to have appropriate expectations when they are considering surgery for stress incontinence. Those with persistent or worsening OAB following surgery can be quite disappointed. Many refractory mixed patients are best served with a third-line OAB therapy but need to realize that the SUI will persist.

Reassessing the stress component

Reassessment of the SUI component and clarifying the patient's expectations is important to direct future therapy. What we mean by this is to reevaluate the severity of the SUI and its relative contribution to the mixed presentation, as well as its importance to the individual. Subsequently, a sling or third-line OAB therapy can be more easily justified.

We review the history, physical, and urodynamic findings to determine how severe is the stress incontinence in each individual. A patient with mild SUI noted in the history and physical examination and with a leak point pressure of 135 cmH$_2$O is different than a mixed patient with severe stress symptoms, a high volume positive cough test, and impressive urodynamic ISD. This reassessment of the stress component can assist the clinician in recommending treatment options. When a patient says that she can "live with her stress incontinence" and is more bothered by her overactive bladder, she has just helped you in prescribing her individual diagnosis to treatment pathway.

Individual diagnosis to treatment pathway for Wendy (A–D)

Wendy (A–D) have mixed incontinence with varying urodynamic findings. Let's discuss their respected diagnosis to treatment pathway based on the evaluation.

Wendy (A)

Wendy (A) will be treated with medical and behavioral therapy. In spite of her normal filling cystometry, she does have an overactive bladder. She has moderately severe ISD, but may still reach her treatment goal with conservative therapies. As previously mentioned, there are a number of advantages to an initial non-surgical approach.

- Based on her moderately severe urgency incontinence, we would try a number of OAB agents but not hesitate to recommend a sling. We can appreciate those who may advance to surgery more expeditiously.
- If and when Wendy (A) is treated surgically, we would counsel her according to the index mixed patient template. Her cystometric bladder storage characteristics are favorable, and we have no increased concern that her OAB will persist or worsen postoperatively.

Wendy (B)

Wendy (B) clearly has unfavorable storage characteristics combined with mild urodynamic SUI. She will be aggressively managed with medical and behavioral therapy and only offered surgery after a number of agents have been utilized.

- If Wendy (B) fails medication, her SUI component and expectations will be reassessed in order to better advance her treatment pathway. Based on that discussion, either a sling or third-line OAB therapy will be recommended.

  If Wendy (B) is considering a sling, the index mixed patient template will be modified based on her urodynamics and unfavorable bladder storage characteristics. We would emphasize our concern that she may have persistent or worsening storage symptoms postoperatively. The existence of third-line OAB treatments would be mentioned as part of her sling consent process. Urethral bulking agents are a good option to consider in this population hoping to avoid an unhappy sling patient.

- In contrast, if Wendy (B) can live with her SUI, she will be offered a refractory OAB therapy. We'll speak further about third-line treatments in another diagnosis to treatment module.

Wendy (C)

- Wendy (C) has moderately severe urgency and stress incontinence based on her comprehensive evaluation. We would treat her like Wendy (B), recognizing she likely will need a sling or bulking agent if her SUI remains bothersome in spite of medical and behavioral therapy. Because of her unfavorable storage characteristics, the surgical index template will similarly be modified and future third-line OAB therapies mentioned.

Wendy (D)

- Wendy (D) has unfavorable bladder storage characteristics and no urodynamic SUI. If she fails medical and behavioral therapy, she will be offered a third-line OAB treatment. It would be difficult to justify a sling in her circumstance.

- If she continued to be bothered by SUI after a refractory OAB therapy, we would then recommend a urethral bulking agent over a sling, although both are options.

Case 1 / Patient with moderate stress and urgency incontinence

We presented a single patient with stress and urgency incontinence and demonstrated how urodynamics can identify four unique individuals, with each one sitting in different locations along the mixed spectrum altering their diagnosis to treatment pathway. But the variability and complexity between individual mixed patients is often much greater than this single case.

A woman with flooding urgency incontinence, hourly frequency, and who leaks a small amount playing tennis and soaking 8 pads per day will be managed differently from one who wears two liners to manage her SUI and rare urgency incontinence. Urodynamic findings in these patients can vary significantly once again influencing their diagnosis to treatment pathway.

Pelvic Organ Prolapse (POP): Diagnosis to Treatment Pathway

The prevalence of symptomatic pelvic organ prolapse (POP) ranges from 4% to 12% and the estimated lifetime risk of a woman having surgery for POP or incontinence is 11.1%. Urodynamics is recommended as part of the preoperative assessment, since many of these patients have associated lower urinary tract symptoms that can often be addressed simultaneously. A thorough preoperative evaluation also helps educate patients and establish appropriate treatment expectations.

This module addresses the use of urodynamics in the evaluation of lower urinary tract function in the presence of surgical prolapse, and how the study results can impact the diagnosis to treatment pathway. It concentrates on the assessment of how incompetent the outlet is and whether or not the SUI should be addressed during surgery How well the bladder stores and the assessment of voiding efficiency is factored into the decision process.

The AUA/SUFU adult urodynamic guideline statements for women with stress urinary incontinence and overactive bladder also apply to prolapse patients who concomitantly have these lower urinary tract symptoms.

Guidelines

Specific to prolapse, clinicians should perform stress testing with reduction of the prolapse in women with high grade pelvic organ prolapse (POP) but without the symptom of SUI. Multi-channel urodynamics with prolapse reduction may be used to assess for occult stress incontinence and detrusor dysfunction in these women with associated LUTS.

Occult SUI is defined as stress incontinence observed only after the reduction of co-existent prolapse. A significant proportion of women with high grade POP who do not have the symptom of SUI will be found to have occult SUI.

Prolapse can be reduced with a number of tools including but not limited to a pessary, a ring forceps or a vaginal pack (Figure M4-1). Reduction of the prolapse can be done independently or during urodynamic testing.

Multi-channel UDS can also assess for the presence of detrusor dysfunction in women with high grade POP. Some patients with high grade POP may have an elevated PVR or be in urinary retention. UDS with the POP reduced can facilitate evaluation of detrusor function and determine if the elevated PVR/retention is due to detrusor underactivity, outlet obstruction or a combination of both.

Invasive UDS may be performed both with and without reduction of the POP to evaluate bladder function. This may be helpful in the prediction of postoperative bladder function once the POP has been surgically repaired.

We perform stress testing with and without the prolapse reduced during physical examination and with urodynamics. The latter has the advantage of ensuring that the bladder is full when SUI is assessed. The degree of urethral hypermobility, severity of leakage, and LPP's are evaluated.

Urodynamics may identify the presence of unfavorable bladder storage characteristics in POP patients with OAB or mixed stress and urgency incontinence. Prolapse patients may have elevated residuals secondary to an obstructing cystocele hinging over the bladder neck, especially in the case of prior stress incontinence surgery, or from poor bladder contractility. Pressure flow urodynamics with and without the prolapse reduced can differentiate the two and help predict postoperative voiding efficiency.

Figure M4-1: Fluoro study of prolapse and prolapse reduced with forceps

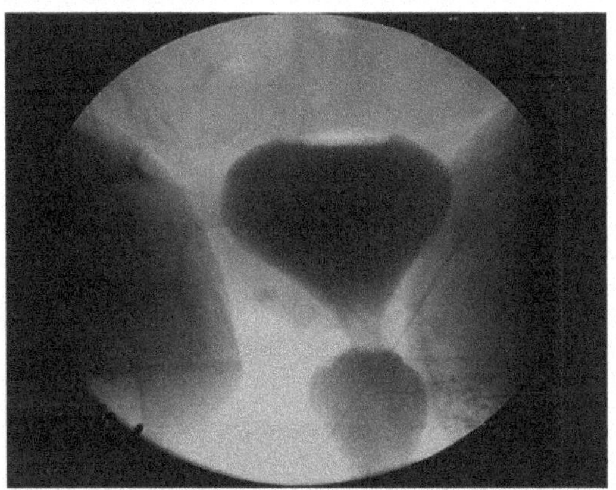

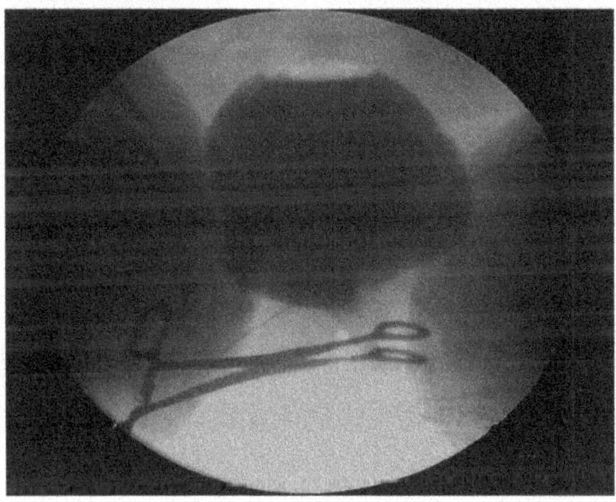

CASE 1

Index Patient with Pelvic Organ Prolapse and Occult SUI

Diagnosis

History

Sharon is a 71-year-old woman with a four year history of symptomatic prolapse. She reports vaginal bulging that is uncomfortable, especially while sitting. She sometimes reduces her prolapse to assist voiding.

She is continent but has mild urinary urgency. She voids every one to two hours and has no nocturia. She has a slower flow but feels empty after urination.

She has had a hysterectomy and has minimal medical comorbidities. Her prolapse symptoms are significantly impacting her quality of life.

Sharon has symptomatic POP and minimal voiding dysfunction. She has mild overactive bladder and voiding symptoms. She is considering prolapse surgery and urodynamics were recommended.

Physical exam

On pelvic examination the patient has a moderate size cystocele that just reaches the introitus. She has a central defect and her vaginal cuff is reasonably well supported. She has no posterior prolapse. During coughing, she has moderate urethral and bladder neck hypermobility, and leaked a small amount only with the cystocele reduced.

Post-void residual urine volume

43 mL

Urinalysis

Rare bacteria, few WBC's, 0 RBC's

Urodynamics

Sharon (A)

During urodynamics, the patient had a MCC of 462 mL with normal bladder sensation. During filling, she had no detrusor overactivity. She had moderately severe urodynamic SUI with or without the prolapse reduced with a LPP of 51 cmH$_2$O at 300 mL. During voiding her P$_{det}$max was 21 cmH$_2$O and the Qmax was 18 mL/sec. The flow pattern was normal and her EMG activity silenced during voiding.

Sharon (B)

During urodynamics, the patient had a hyposensitive bladder with a MCC of 930 mL. She had infrequent low pressure detrusor overactivity associated with mild urgency. She leaked a few drops at 800 mL with a LPP of 147 cmH$_2$O. During voiding, she did not generate a detrusor contraction and strained to urinate. Her flow was intermittent with a Qmax was 10 mL/sec. EMG activity increased with straining, and she emptied efficiently.

Sharon (C)

During urodynamics, the patient had a MCC of 262 mL and increased bladder sensation. Cystometry demonstrated multiple detrusor contractions reaching a pressure of 16 cmH$_2$O and associated with moderate urgency incontinence. She had small volume urodynamic SUI with a LPP of 132 cmH$_2$O. With and without the prolapse reduced, she had difficulty voiding in the lab setting. After relaxing and water running, she voided 200 mL with a P$_{det}$max of 5 cmH$_2$O and a Qmax of 6 mL/sec. The detrusor contraction was poorly sustained, and her flow pattern was prolonged. EMG activity increased during voiding. She reported that the void was representative of her normal (Figure M4-2).

Figure M4-2: Sharon (C) urodynamics

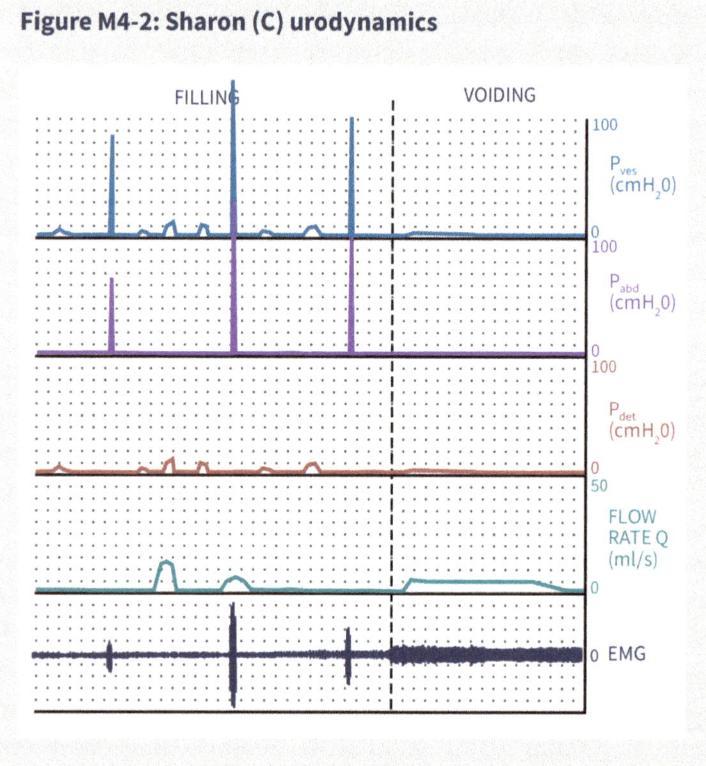

Diagnosis

Sharon (A-C) have pelvic organ prolapse with mild overactive bladder and flow symptoms. They have mild SUI on physical examination with their prolapse reduced.

Sharon (A)

Sharon (A) has normal filling cystometry and moderately severe urodynamic SUI. Her urodynamics reconfirm the presence of her having occult stress urinary incontinence. She generates a good detrusor contraction during voiding and empties efficiently.

Sharon (B)

Sharon (B) has a large capacity hyposensitive bladder with low pressure detrusor overactivity. She has mild urodynamic SUI with a high LPP leaking a few drops at high bladder volumes. During voiding she does not generate a detrusor contraction and strains to urinate.

With further questioning, Sharon (B) reconfirms straining to void. She often uses positional changes and a Credé maneuver to assist voiding.

Sharon (C)

Sharon (C) has significantly reduced bladder capacity associated with detrusor overactivity and moderately severe urgency incontinence. She has unfavorable bladder storage characteristics in combination with mild urodynamic SUI.

During voiding, Sharon (C) generates a poorly sustained weak detrusor contraction and has pelvic floor dyssynergia. She subsequently reports difficulty voiding in public and has urinary hesitancy. Her flow sometimes stops and starts but she does feel empty after urination.

Diagnosis to treatment pathway

Sharon (A-C)'s diagnosis to treatment pathway is influenced by their urodynamics. Before discussing each one, we would like to make a few additional comments regarding prolapse patients.

Patient selection

We consider treating stress incontinence in three types of patients who are planning to have surgery for pelvic organ prolapse. These include those who report stress incontinence, as well as patients who demonstrate occult SUI on physical examination or during urodynamics. If any of these three occur, a "SUI discussion" is warranted.

Many patients with occult SUI when left untreated don't leak following prolapse surgery. The stress test is good but it doesn't necessarily represent the patient's natural postoperative vesicourethral function. Assessing how incompetent the outlet is helps predict whether a patient may leak or not after surgery. A woman who has high volume occult SUI on physical examination and during urodynamics has a LPP of 32 cmH_2O is more likely to be incontinent versus one who leaks a few drops with a hard cough and has a high leak point pressure.

We don't recommend a stress incontinence procedure to patients not having subjective or objective SUI regardless of the degree of prolapse. Some data suggests that those with high grade POP should undergo a "prophylactic sling" but we don't concur. In our experience, the rate of de novo SUI is low and doesn't justify this more aggressive approach which has its own morbidities including the potential for obstruction and de novo detrusor overactivity.

An additional group that needs consideration are POP patients with detrusor overactivity but who do not have urgency incontinence. Their urinary loss may be prevented by the 'kink' at the bladder neck from the cystocele especially if the patient has had prior incontinence surgery. Surgical correction of the cystocele could unmask their urgency incontinence. This group is most troublesome if their postoperative OAB does not respond to medication.

Patient factors

Remember that there are a number of factors to consider when recommending surgery for SUI. How incompetent is the outlet, how well does the bladder store, voiding efficiency, and patient features and expectations are important aspects of the evaluation and post urodynamic discussion.

There is an association between pelvic organ prolapse and overactive bladder. The incidence of detrusor overactivity increases with the degree of prolapse and may be related to pelvic floor neuropraxia. Many POP patients have unfavorable bladder storage characteristics demonstrated on cystometry even in the absence of significant OAB symptoms.

Be cognizant of the elderly patient who has significant bladder and vaginal vault prolapse. Many of them have a large-capacity poorly contractile detrusor with a tendency toward inefficient bladder emptying. They are at higher risk of developing urinary retention following pelvic floor reconstruction and a sling.

A significant number of POP patients are willing to live with their baseline incontinence as long as their bothersome prolapse is effectively managed. Many have medical co-morbidities or risk factors for neurogenic bladder and are prone to having persistent voiding dysfunction following a sling. Liberally offering a procedure for SUI to many of these patients may not be the best diagnosis to treatment strategy.

Staged therapy

The incidence of de novo or worsening SUI following prolapse surgery is low. Rarely, it can be severe and patients need to be aware of this possibility. Soaking several pads daily after successful pelvic floor reconstruction in a patient who was previously continent or had mild incontinence can be upsetting.

The good news for those experiencing postoperative SUI is that it can be effectively managed with pelvic floor muscle retraining or a subsequent bladder neck suspension or bulking agent. Aware of this option, many patients elect a conservative approach avoiding the risks of a sling that in most cases is not necessary. The preoperative discussion of the possibility of having de novo or worsening SUI that can be managed by staged therapy should be documented in the medical record.

Individual diagnosis to treatment pathway for Sharon (A–C)

Sharon (A)

Sharon (A) represents the index POP patient with occult SUI demonstrated on physical examination and during urodynamics. She has mild lower urinary tract symptoms and favorable bladder storage and emptying characteristics.

- Her urodynamic SUI is moderately severe, and we would recommend a sling or bulking agent. Based on her urodynamic findings, we would not change our usual preoperative surgical discussion.

  Sharon (A) should realize that a sling is not a benign procedure. From her perspective being dry after surgery is no different than her preoperative status. She will likely view experiencing any postoperative voiding dysfunction, urinary incontinence, or sling complication very unfavorably. Taking on surgical risk "to be the same" in an attempt to prevent something that may or may not happen can be the beginning an unpleasant downward and slippery slope.

  Sharon (A) must also understand that slings fail. In patients destined to develop de novo SUI, at least 10% will still do so in spite of having a sling. Waking up with de novo stress or urgency urinary incontinence is always a possibility.

Sharon (B)

- Based on urodynamics, we will encourage Sharon (B) not to have a concomitant bladder neck suspension to treat her occult SUI. She has a large capacity poorly contractile bladder, placing her at higher risk for postoperative urinary retention. If her occult SUI were addressed, we would recommend a bulking agent. Her chances of developing postoperative SUI are low, and it can be managed with staged therapy.

Sharon (C)

- Sharon (C) has complicated underlying bladder dysfunction. Recommending whether or not her occult SUI should be simultaneously treated is difficult. A sling can upset her baseline bladder dysfunction and a conservative approach is wise.

  She has mild urinary frequency but unfavorable bladder storage characteristics on urodynamics. With or without a sling, she is at risk of having persistent or worsening overactive bladder postoperatively. In addition, her history and urodynamics support the presence of pelvic floor dysfunction. Poor pelvic floor relaxation during voiding, in combination with her weak detrusor, likely places her at higher risk of retention with a sling. A urethral bulking agent may be a better option.

The guidelines suggest that a positive physical examination is sufficient to diagnose occult SUI. But how would we identify both Sharon (B) and (C) who are clearly not an index POP patient? These three Sharons are very different and should be managed with their own diagnosis to treatment pathway. Once again, the patient's complexity is only realized by routinely performing urodynamics.

CASE 2

Pelvic Organ Prolapse with Elevated PVR

Diagnosis

History

Libby is a 61-year-old woman with a two year history of symptomatic prolapse. She reports vaginal bulging and splinting to assist voiding.

The patient voids every two to three hours and gets up once during the night to urinate. She has a markedly reduced flow and does not feel empty after urination. She has no urinary incontinence.

Libby has recurrent UTI's and has had a hysterectomy. She has minimal medical comorbidities and is reasonably active. She is bothered by both her prolapse and flow symptoms.

Libby has symptomatic POP and significant flow symptoms. She has mild urinary frequency and a history of recurrent UTI's. She was evaluated with urodynamics and cystoscopy.

Physical exam

On pelvic examination, the patient has a large cystocele that extends 2 cm beyond the introitus. Her vaginal cuff descends approximately 4 cm. She has no posterior prolapse. During coughing, she has mild urethral hypermobility and no incontinence with and without the prolapse reduced.

Post-void residual urine volume

179 mL

Urinalysis

Rare bacteria, few WBC's, 0 RBC's

Cystoscopy

Normal cystoscopy with no intravesical or urethral abnormalities.

Urodynamics

Libby (A)

During urodynamics, the patient had a MCC of 510 mL with normal bladder sensation. She had no detrusor overactivity or urodynamic SUI. During voiding, she voided 300 mL with a P_{det}max of 41 cmH$_2$O and a Qmax was 8 mL/sec. Her PVR was greater than 200 mL. With the prolapse reduced, her repeat pressure flow analysis normalized and her PVR was zero. EMG activity was normal. (Figure M4-3).

Figure M4-3: Libby (A) urodynamics

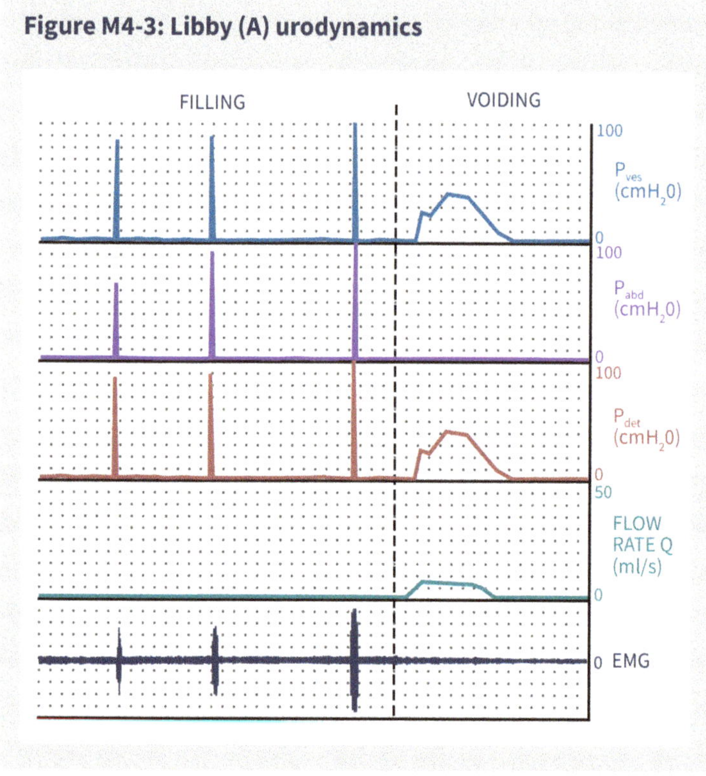

Libby (B)

During urodynamics the patient had a MCC of 651 mL with mild decreased bladder sensation. During filling, she had no detrusor overactivity or urodynamic SUI. With and without the prolapse reduced, she voided 400 mL with a P_{det}max of 7 cmH$_2$O and a Qmax was 8 mL/sec. Her PVR was approximately 250 mL. EMG activity was normal.

Libby (C)

During urodynamics, the patient had a MCC of 558 mL. She had normal bladder sensation and no detrusor overactivity. After reducing the prolapse at 500 mL, she had mild to moderate urodynamic SUI with a LPP of 76 cmH$_2$O. With the prolapse reduced, she voided 460 mL with a P_{det}max of 18 cmH$_2$O and a Qmax of 16 mL/sec. Her EMG activity was normal and her PVR was 90 mL.

Diagnosis

Libby (A–C) have symptomatic POP and bothersome flow symptoms. They have a feeling of incomplete bladder emptying and an elevated residual. They have a history of recurrent UTI's.

Libby (A)

Libby (A) has normal bladder filling and no urodynamic SUI. She has an obstructing cystocele with an elevated PVR. Her pressure-flow study and ability to empty normalized with prolapse reduction.

Libby (B)

Libby (B) has a reasonably large bladder associated with mild decreased sensation. Her inefficient emptying is secondary to a poorly contractile bladder and not pelvic organ prolapse. Reducing her cystocele had no bearing on her ability to empty.

Libby (C)

Libby (C) has normal bladder filling and mild to moderate occult urodynamic SUI. With her prolapse reduced, her residual improved but was still mildly elevated. Her voiding parameters otherwise were reasonably normal.

Diagnosis to treatment pathway

Libby (A–C) have pelvic organ prolapse with flow symptoms and elevated post-void residuals. UTI's secondary to incomplete bladder emptying still respond favorably to prophylactic antibiotics.

Libby (A)

- Libby (A) will be offered pelvic floor reconstruction to address her prolapse and voiding issues. Although her urodynamics identify an obstructing cystocele, she will be cautioned about the possibility of still having an elevated PVR postoperatively. Voiding efficiency relies on a number of factors and surgical guarantees are unwise. Her recurrent UTI's may also persist if they are due to chronic perineal colonization and not elevated PVR's.

Libby (B)

- We would recommend Libby (B) prolapse surgery to address her symptomatic prolapse but not her bothersome flow. Her slow flow and incomplete emptying appears to be secondary to a poorly contractile bladder and not an obstructing cystocele. The prolapse repair may help her voiding, but this should not be her expectation. Alpha-adrenergic antagonists and pelvic floor therapy can sometimes be effective.

Libby (C)

- Based on urodynamics, Libby (C)'s bothersome prolapse and voiding may also benefit from pelvic floor surgery. Her PVR definitely improved with reduction of the prolapse, and surgery could yield similar benefit.
- Libby (C) has mild to moderate occult urodynamic SUI, but we don't recommend a sling. Even though her PVR is expected to improve with a cystocele repair, her risk of retention is still concerning. For those more bullish regarding management of her occult SUI, we would recommend a bulking agent.
- If Libby (C) developed de novo SUI, it could be effectively managed with a second procedure. Her voiding efficiency would then be apparent and a sling might be an excellent treatment option.

Post-Sling Voiding Dysfunction: Diagnosis to Treatment Pathway

Many female patients with voiding dysfunction have had a previous sling or bladder neck suspension. When causal, the patient typically develops de novo or worsening lower urinary tract symptoms soon after surgery. This important temporal relationship differentiates them from those having persistent or a new onset of unrelated symptoms. If a patient who voids normally prior to a stress incontinence procedure acutely voids abnormally after the operation, the surgery is likely the cause. However, preoperative and postoperative urodynamics, if available, can help to better understand the underlying causes of the problem.

There is a natural tendency for patients to report that their symptoms started after surgery when in fact the two are not related, especially if the surgery was done in the distant past. A clinical assessment of bladder function before and after surgery is important, since it could have diagnostic consequences. The historical facts become less clear when the surgery was performed years prior.

In the case of an obstructing sling, it may take years for the obstruction to secondarily upset normal bladder filling and emptying, making a causal diagnosis difficult. Many patients develop idiopathic voiding dysfunction unrelated to previous events.

Urinary retention, obstructive voiding, overactive bladder, pelvic pain, or persistent SUI weeks or years following a sling can be very disappointing to both patient and provider. Patient expectations are high, the presentation can be complex, and a second surgery may not be the answer.

We believe that a thorough evaluation is warranted in this challenging population of patients. We will present a number of cases emphasizing patient complexity, and how urodynamics can help in recommending effective diagnosis to treatment pathways.

CASE 1

The Index Post-Sling Voiding Dysfunction Patient

Diagnosis

History

Gabby is a 66-year-old woman who reports a poor floor and feeling of incomplete bladder emptying since her sling six weeks prior. Her flow stops and starts, and sometimes she leans back in order to urinate.

Her urinary frequency has worsened, and she is now voiding every 30–60 minutes associated with urgency. She no longer has SUI but has had a few episodes of urgency incontinence.

Her voiding dysfunction is significantly impacting her quality of life. Prior to surgery her flow was reasonable, and she did not require positional maneuvers. She used to void every 1–2 hours and had mild urgency that was not bothersome. She was using 3 pads daily for SUI. She is upset about her changed voiding function and wonders if the mesh is the problem.

Gabby has no other complicating urologic factors and minimal medical comorbidities. She was treated elsewhere and did not have preoperative urodynamics. She was told that her residual was normal prior to surgery.

Gabby has worsening flow and OAB symptoms since her sling. She has traded her SUI for worsening urinary urgency and infrequent urgency incontinence. The symptoms are significantly impacting her quality of life, and she is displeased with her surgical outcome. She was evaluated with urodynamics and cystoscopy.

Physical exam

On pelvic examination, the patient has mild urethral and bladder neck hypermobility and no SUI. She has no prolapse or evidence of sling extrusion. All incisions are healed, and she has no vaginal or perineal tenderness.

Post-void residual urine volume

168 mL

Urinalysis

Normal

Cystoscopy

The patient's cystoscopic evaluation was normal. There was no mesh erosion or obvious signs of urethral obstruction. She had no pain during filling or evidence of cystitis.

Diagnosis

Gabby is an index patient with bladder outlet obstruction secondary to a sling. She no longer has SUI but has worsening voiding and storage symptoms associated with an elevated post-void residual.

Before recommending her diagnosis to treatment pathway we would like to discuss this population. The diagnosis of post-sling obstruction can be challenging, and a thorough stepwise approach is recommended. An unsuccessful release of a sling can further complicate an already difficult situation.

The development of de novo voiding or storage symptoms immediately after surgery strongly supports the diagnosis. Many patients report poor flow, hesitancy, stopping and starting, and/or a feeling of incomplete emptying. Obstructed patients often void small amounts and have elevated residuals.

OAB can be secondary to obstruction or from incomplete bladder emptying. The latter is especially the case in patients with low functional capacities. It is well established that approximately 1–2% of patients develop de novo or worsening OAB following a bladder neck suspension in the absence of any identifiable cause. Also the ability to hold more urine following a successful sling may sometimes unmask an occult urgent bladder.

On physical examination, it's important to look for associated complications or findings that could be relevant. These include the presence of vaginal mesh extrusion or local pain and tenderness causing pelvic floor dyssynergia.

Sometimes, it's apparent that the sling has been placed at the level of the proximal urethra and bladder neck versus the mid-urethra, which can be more obstructing. The anterior vaginal wall may be elevated at the location of the sling. The presence of a small cystocele hinging over a fixed urethra is also suggestive. This hinging effect may be more pronounced when the patient sits to urinate (Figure M5-1).

Figure M5-1: Mesh sling identified under the proximal urethra with hinging cystocele during urethrolysis.

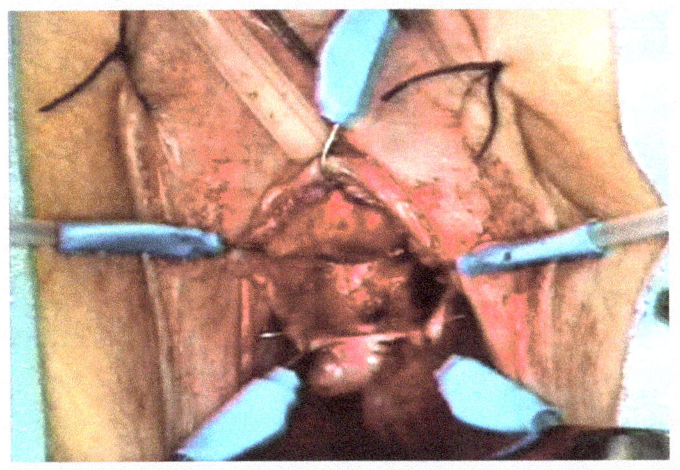

Prior to the advent of mid-urethral slings, many obstructed patients had significant elevation of the urethro-vesical angle on physical exam. The presence of this over-correction shelf was especially common following an open colposuspension and perhaps less so with a pubovaginal sling (Figure M5-2).

Figure M5-2: Significant elevation of the urethro-vesical angle

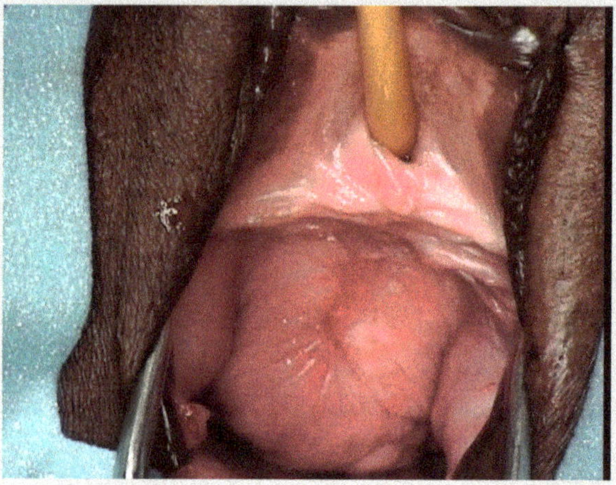

A urinalysis and culture are important in the assessment. Microscopic hematuria could suggest sling erosion and patients commonly have UTI's postoperatively.

When obstructed, the uroflow pattern is generally depressed and prolonged or intermittent secondary to straining. The post-void residual is often elevated, but a normal PVR does not rule out the presence of obstruction.

Cystoscopy is recommended to diagnose mesh erosion into the bladder or urethra. Sometimes, the location of obstruction can be appreciated endoscopically. An elevated ski-jump effect at the bladder neck may be a sign of overcorrection.

Urodynamics should be liberally performed in this population. The presence of high pressure and low flow voiding helps confirm the diagnosis, but is often absent, even when obstructed, because many female patients don't generate strong enough detrusor contractions to produce high pressure voiding. Having said that, a normal pressure and well sustained contraction in the face of a poor flow and elevated residual is highly suggestive of obstruction.

The presence of a large capacity poorly contractile bladder is an important finding. It may be causing the flow symptoms versus an obstructing sling. A lack of pelvic floor coordination may similarly be an aggravating factor.

Unfavorable bladder storage characteristics may be identified and clinically relevant, especially in those considering release of a sling. Detrusor overactivity may be due to obstruction, but, in many cases, is unrelated and could persist following a urethrolysis.

Diagnosis to treatment pathway

We believe that Gabby is obstructed and doesn't necessarily need urodynamics. Her abrupt change in voiding function with a clear picture of her "before and after" strongly support the diagnosis, and we would recommend to release her sling.

Considerations before releasing a sling

The best time to cut a sling is controversial. We tend to wait 4–6 weeks with synthetic slings, and 12 weeks or longer following non-mesh procedures. Timing is influenced by the severity of symptoms and the patient's willingness to allow time for improvement. Complete urinary retention two weeks post-sling in an anxious patient probably needs to be addressed more acutely than a patient who is coping well as her symptoms and PVR slowly improve. Whether or not the patient has to perform CIC also affects the decision.

Waiting at least four weeks allows the mesh to anchor itself to the endopelvic fascia, providing support at this level. A subsequent mesh incision then effectively converts the sling to a Burch-like procedure which may be adequate to maintain continence.

Whether to cut the mesh at 6 o'clock—or 5 or 7 o'clock to avoid urethral damage (sling incision)—or to cut and partially excise it to the level of the pelvic floor (sling excision) remains controversial. We advise the latter when efficient emptying at all costs is the primary goal of the procedure.

Bladder response to sling incision

When recommending sling incision, the patient should understand how each of her bothersome symptoms may respond. Having appropriate expectations is important, and the discussion should be documented.

The literature supports that 20–30% of patients who undergo vaginal urethrolysis redevelop stress urinary incontinence. We agree, but individualize this prediction based on the patient's pre-sling urethral function. For example, a SUI patient who prior to a sling was soaking 6 pads per day with a leak point pressure of 20 cmH_2O is much more likely to leak postoperatively than one who wore one liner and had a LPP of 140 cmH_2O. Cutting and converting the sling to a Burch-like procedure has a good chance of maintaining continence in the second patient. Dry rates may also be fractionally higher following sling incision versus sling excision.

Beware when releasing the mesh in a continent woman who had significant mixed incontinence prior to her sling. The urethrolysis may not only cause SUI, but she may also experience high volume urgency incontinence.

Being an index patient, we would predict that Gabby's rate of developing SUI with sling incision is approximately 20–30%. Prior to surgery, she had mild SUI and OAB. Her flow symptoms and PVR should improve in the majority of cases. Even though her poor flow appears to be due to obstruction, you can never guarantee success.

When a sling is released, its impact on OAB symptoms is less predictable. Many patients have an undiagnosed chronic overactive bladder that will likely persist following urethrolysis. Long-term bladder outlet obstruction can cause bladder overactivity that may remain postoperatively. When urinary frequency is due to an elevated PVR, it should improve following successful surgery.

Some surgeons offer a second bladder neck suspension at the time of sling incision. We don't recommend this in the midst of treating a complication. We believe that it's best to tackle one problem at a time, and to avoid confusing issues that can occur by placing a second sling if problems persist after the intervention.

CASE 2

Voiding Dysfunction One Year Post-Sling

Diagnosis

History

Jennifer is a 76-year-old woman who reports worsening frequency and bothersome flow symptoms since a sling one year prior. She has no SUI but experiences urgency and then sits for several moments only to void a small amount. Her flow stops and starts, and she doesn't feel empty after urination.

She has hourly frequency and gets up twice during the night to void. She has urgency incontinence with key in the door syndrome and uses one to two pads daily to control her incontinence. Her OAB is having an impact on her quality of life.

Prior to surgery, her flow was good and she felt empty after urination. She had no hesitancy but sometimes strained to urinate. She use to void every one to two hours due to urgency but had no nocturia or urgency incontinence. She had moderately severe SUI requiring three pads per day. She believes that there is something wrong with the mesh and wants it removed.

Jennifer has no other complicating urologic factors and has minimal medical comorbidities. There is no documentation of prior urodynamics or residual urine volume.

Jennifer has worsening flow and OAB symptoms since her sling. Her surgery addressed her SUI but she now has bothersome voiding dysfunction. It has had an impact on her quality of life, and she is concerned about the mesh. She was evaluated with urodynamics and cystoscopy.

Physical exam

On pelvic examination, the patient has mild urethral and bladder neck hypermobility and no SUI. She has no prolapse or evidence of sling extrusion. She has no vaginal or perineal tenderness.

Post-void residual urine volume

168 mL

Urinalysis

Normal

Cystoscopy

Normal

Urodynamics

Jennifer (A)

During urodynamics, the patient had a MCC of 466 mL associated with mild increased bladder sensation. She had no involuntary detrusor overactivity or urodynamic SUI. During pressure flow, her P_{det}max was 52 cmH$_2$O and the Qmax was 8 mL/sec. The flow pattern was depressed and prolonged. EMG activity was normal and the PVR was 153 mL (Figure M5-3).

Figure M5-3: Jennifer (A) Urodynamics

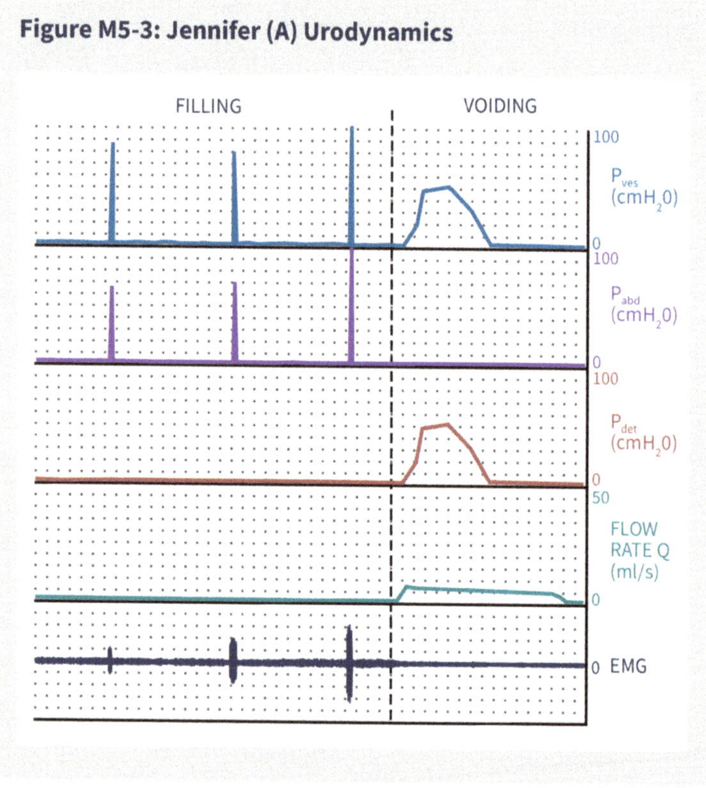

Jennifer (B)

During urodynamics, the patient had a MCC of 222 mL associated with increased bladder sensation. She had impressive involuntary detrusor overactivity reaching pressures of 39 cmH$_2$O associated with mild urgency incontinence. She had no urodynamic SUI. During voiding, she generated a well sustained detrusor contraction with a P$_{det}$max of 22 cmH$_2$O and a Qmax of 4 mL/sec. The flow pattern was depressed and prolonged. EMG activity was normal and the PVR was 142 mL (Figure M5-4).

Figure M5-4: Jennifer (B) Urodynamics

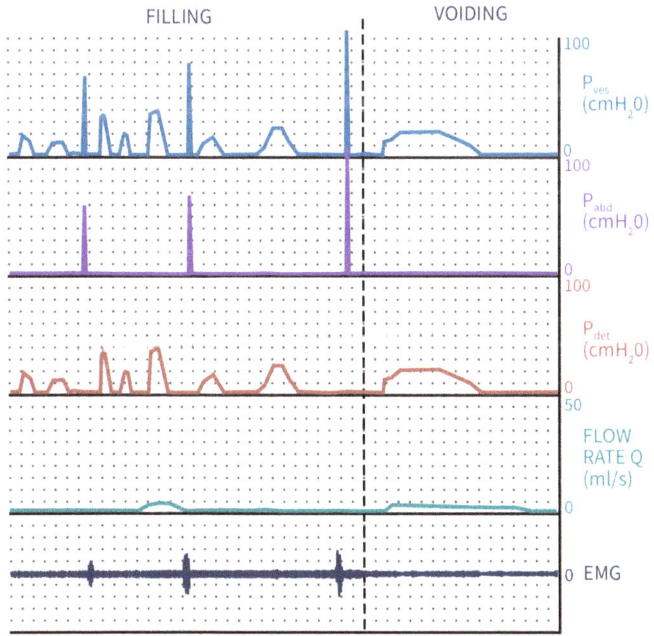

Jennifer (C)

During urodynamics, the patient had a MCC of 963 mL and decreased bladder sensation. She had moderate urgency associated with involuntary detrusor overactivity reaching pressures of 8 cmH$_2$O. She had no urodynamic SUI. During voiding, she did not generate a detrusor contraction and strained to urinate. Her Qmax was 12 mL/sec and her flow pattern was intermittent. Her EMG increased with straining and her PVR was 180 mL (Figure M5-5).

Figure M5–5: Jennifer (C) Urodynamics

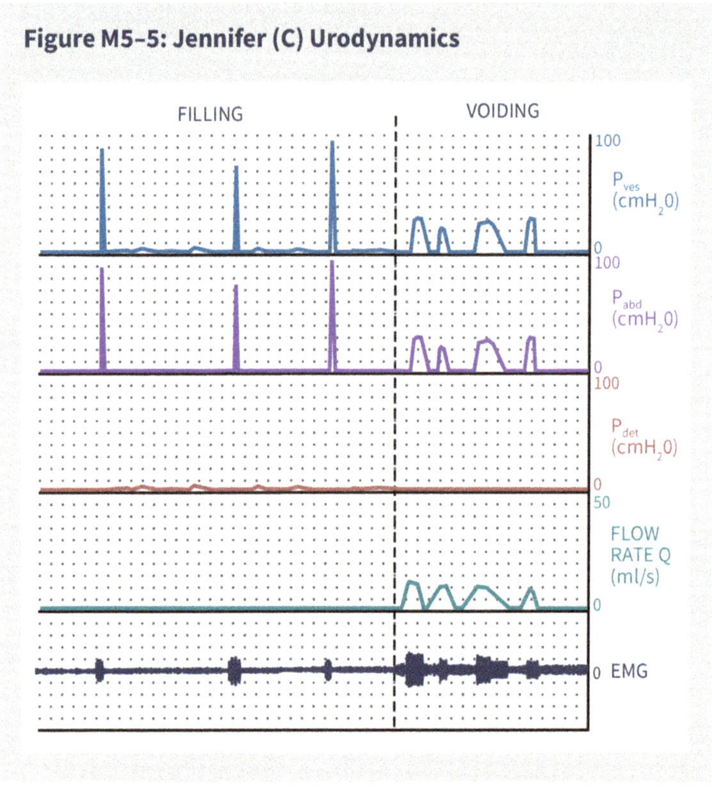

Diagnosis

Jennifer (A-C) have worsening flow and OAB symptoms since their sling. They have incomplete bladder emptying with moderately elevated PVR's. Their symptoms are significantly impacting their quality of life.

Jennifer (A)

Jennifer (A) has normal filling cystometry and no urodynamic SUI. She is obstructed on urodynamics with incomplete bladder emptying.

Jennifer (B)

Jennifer (B) has a markedly reduced bladder capacity and detrusor overactivity. She has unfavorable bladder storage characteristics and no urodynamic SUI. Her pressure flow in combination with an elevated PVR is less definitive but does support the diagnosis of obstruction.

Jennifer (C)

Jennifer (C) has a large capacity bladder associated with decreased bladder sensation. She has low pressure detrusor overactivity and no urodynamic SUI. She does not generate a voluntary detrusor contraction and voids by abdominal straining. Her elevated residual is worsened or caused by her poor detrusor function.

Diagnosis to treatment pathway

Jennifer (A–C) have complicated voiding dysfunction, and their urodynamic findings have an impact on their individual diagnosis to treatment pathway. To some degree, their treatment overlaps with DHIC patients.

We would recommend Jennifer (A–C) a trial of behavioral and pelvic floor therapy and alpha-adrenergic antagonists. A minority of patients respond, avoiding the risk of surgery. A conservative approach gives time to build a relationship with the patient and to establish realistic expectations.

Alpha-blockers improve flow, but they can help OAB by their receptor effects in the dome of the bladder and central nervous system. Improving bladder emptying may also secondarily benefit overactive bladder.

Jennifer (A–C) could be managed with OAB medication. The goal is to control their OAB symptoms while accepting their elevated PVR and bothersome flow. As is the case with traditional DHIC patients, their risk of developing urinary retention is low.

Jennifer (A)

- Jennifer (A) is an excellent candidate for sling incision to treat her voiding dysfunction. Based on urodynamics, her flow symptoms and PVR are likely to improve by releasing the obstruction.
- She has favorable bladder storage characteristics, optimizing her OAB prognosis. Although her OAB will likely respond, some of her symptoms may persist or even worsen. It's important for her to remember that she did have mild OAB prior to surgery. OAB medication that failed prior to urethrolysis can sometimes be effective postoperatively.
- Prior to her sling, Jennifer (A) reported having moderately severe stress incontinence. It is reasonable to predict that the chances of her developing SUI following sling incision is approximately 20–30%. Patients who are continent early after sling lysis are cautioned that their SUI can sometimes return months afterwards.

  If Jennifer (A) is unwilling to accept the risk of developing de novo SUI, we would recommend either sacral nerve stimulation or PTNS to control her OAB if she failed medical therapy. In a lower percentage of patients, neuromodulation may also improve flow and PVR. We prefer fixing the problem by cutting the sling over neuromodulation, but both are treatment options.

Jennifer (B)

- Jennifer (B) is obstructed, and her flow and PVR will likely respond to sling incision. She needs to be aware that she is at higher risk of having persistent or worsening OAB based on her unfavorable bladder storage characteristics demonstrated on urodynamics. Even if her detrusor overactivity is secondary to obstruction, cutting the sling may expose her to significant urgency incontinence. Neuromodulation spares her the risk of developing post-lysis SUI or mixed incontinence.

Jennifer (C)

- Jennifer (C) may not respond as well to releasing the sling. She has a large capacity poorly contractile bladder and may have persistent flow symptoms or an elevated residual postoperatively. She is also at risk of developing de novo SUI or mixed incontinence.

Some of Jennifer (B) and (C)'s storage and voiding issues have likely been present long before their sling surgery. The sling may have worsened or tipped the balance, but it's likely not the only problem. Both are at higher risk of experiencing less favorable outcomes verses an index patient, and they should be consented appropriately.

If Jennifer (A–C) presented five years following a sling, there are additional factors to consider. First, be careful blaming an event that occurred many years prior. Defining the before and after is difficult and fraught with inaccuracy. Time also allows for the development of independent voiding dysfunction secondary to aging or other medical comorbidities. A careful history may reveal that the patient's symptoms worsened more recently and not immediately after surgery.

Case 2 / Voiding dysfunction one year post-sling

Chronic bladder outlet obstruction can cause permanent detrusor changes that may persist long-term after urethrolysis. Some of Jennifer (B) and (C)'s urodynamic findings may be secondary to five years of obstruction. Similar to male LUTS managed by transurethral resection of the prostate, their bladder dysfunction may persist in spite of relieving the obstruction.

We are reluctant to release a sling in patients presenting many years afterwards. Persistent or worsening voiding dysfunction is a real possibility, and patients may redevelop SUI or mixed incontinence which could be severe. Symptomatic management using a combination of behavioral therapy, alpha-blockers, OAB agents, and neuromodulation is recommended. OnabotulinumtoxinA may play a role in those who are willing to perform CIC.

CASE 3

Persistent SUI Following a Sling

Diagnosis

History

Bobby is a 56-year-old woman who has stress incontinence in spite of her having a sling one year prior. She wears two to three pads daily to manage her SUI, which is unchanged from her preoperative status.

She voids every two hours and has no nocturia. Her flow is normal, and she otherwise has minimal voiding dysfunction.

She is disappointed over her persistent incontinence and is seeking further treatment. Bobby has no other complicating urologic factors and has minimal medical comorbidities.

Bobby has SUI and her sling was unsuccessful. She is bothered by her incontinence and was evaluated with cystoscopy and urodynamics.

Physical exam

On pelvic examination, the patient has mild urethral and bladder neck hypermobility and moderate SUI. She has no prolapse or evidence of sling extrusion. She has no vaginal or perineal tenderness.

Post-void residual urine volume

12 mL

Urinalysis

Normal

Cystoscopy

The patient's cystoscopic evaluation was normal. There was no mesh erosion or indications of urethral obstruction. Endoscopically, the urethra was healthy and normal length.

Urodynamics

Bobby (A)

During urodynamics, the patient had a MCC of 526 mL associated with mild increased bladder sensation. During filling, she had no involuntary detrusor overactivity. Her LPP was 112 cmH$_2$O leaking a mild amount. Her pressure flow and EMG were normal.

Bobby (B)

During urodynamics, the patient had a MCC of 526 mL associated with mild increased bladder sensation. During filling, she had no involuntary detrusor overactivity. Her LPP was 11 cmH$_2$O leaking a large amount at low bladder volumes. Her pressure flow and EMG were normal.

Diagnosis

Bobby (A) and (B) have persistent SUI in spite of a previous sling, and their symptoms are impacting their quality of life.

Bobby (A)

- Bobby (A) has normal filling cystometry and no detrusor overactivity. She has mild urodynamic SUI leaking a small amount with a high LPP. Her voiding function is normal.

Bobby (B)

- Bobby (B) has normal filling cystometry and no detrusor overactivity. Her urodynamics demonstrate significant ISD and stress urinary incontinence. Her voiding function is normal.

Diagnosis to treatment pathway

Both Bobby (A) and (B) have stress urinary incontinence, and their urodynamic findings should be considered when recommending their diagnosis to treatment pathway. In addition, the severity of their urethral dysfunction may have prognostic implications.

Bobby (A)

Bobby (A) can be treated like any index SUI patient, offering the various non-surgical and surgical treatments. Even if she declines pelvic floor muscle training, it's wise to document the discussion.

- We would treat Bobby (A) with a second mid-urethral sling or urethral bulking agent. We use a retropubic sling regardless of the initial approach, but, in her case, a trans-obturator is a good option based on her milder urethral dysfunction. The sling is performed like a virginal case, and the initial mesh is left untouched and usually not visualized. We recommend to tension the sling the same as usual, resisting any temptation to make the sling "tighter."

  The literature supports that bladder neck suspensions are successful in treating post-sling SUI. Their efficacy is a bit lower, and we generally predict success in approximately 80% of cases.

Bobby (B)

- Bobby (B) is more complicated because she has significant ISD. We would treat her with a retropubic sling and not a trans-obturator. The presence of severe ISD lowers the success rate of slings by an additional 10%.

Bulking agents are an excellent salvage procedure for Bobby (A) and (B), avoiding the risks and failure rate associated with a second sling. Their pros and cons should be made clear, and promising a cure is ill-advised.

When to use a compressive pubovaginal sling is debatable, but a fixed stovepipe urethra is one of the indications. We concomitantly remove any sub-urethral mesh to avoid it eroding into the urethra now compressed by the second sling. Removing the mesh may also help make the urethra more compressible.

Other factors may exist that complicate the management. A short or scarred urethra may not accommodate a second sling, and bulking agents are preferred. Prior cystoscopy can help assess length, angulation, and healthiness of the urethra. Whether or not it's wise to place the bulking agent away from the mesh avoiding potential erosion is unknown.

Be careful adding a second sling to a patient who may be tending towards poor bladder emptying. These include patients with poor flow, a history of retention, mildly elevated residual, a poorly contractile detrusor, a sling elevating the proximal urethra, and others. Adding on a second sling in these circumstances could tip the balance causing retention, and a bulking agent may be the preferred treatment.

When slings fail, they usually fail early. The patient often reports immediate SUI even if she has not resumed normal activity. Telling patients who are leaking from day one that their continence may improve with healing is usually not in the patient's best interest.

The best time to repeat a sling is not clear, but we generally wait four months before proceeding. We caution against earlier attempts to pull the sling tighter or replace it with a second. Surgical success can never be guaranteed, and it's best to follow good surgical principles and to control expectations.

LUTS Secondary to BPH: Diagnosis to Treatment Pathway

LUTS secondary to BPH affects millions of men, significantly impacting their quality of life. Treatment goals include alleviating symptoms, altering disease progression, and preventing complications. The symptoms are consistent with obstruction (hesitancy, poor flow, incomplete emptying) and storage symptoms (frequency, nocturia, urgency and urgency incontinence).

The majority of patients are managed with behavioral therapy and medication. Pharmacologic classes include alpha-adrenergic antagonists (alpha-blockers), 5-alpha-reductase inhibitors (5-ARIs), phosphodiesterase type-5 inhibitors (PDE5i), antimuscarinics, and β3-agonists. Medications are usually prescribed for bothersome moderate-to-severe symptoms. Regardless of symptom severity, patients not bothered by their lower urinary tract symptoms can be managed with watchful waiting.

Alpha-blockers are the treatment of choice because of their efficacy, tolerability, and speed of onset. 5-ARIs reduce symptoms and lower the risk of acute urinary retention and need for surgery. Tadalafil is approved for male LUTS with or without erectile dysfunction. Antimuscarinics and β3-agonists treat storage symptoms, and all of these agents can be used as monotherapy or in combination.

The surgical options for BPH/BPO continue to increase, including effective and well tolerated office-based procedures. Even robotic assisted surgery is playing an important role. In this module we refer

to all procedures as prostate surgery (outlet resistance reduction procedures), regardless of type.

Guidelines

*The BPH guidelines state that surgery is recommended for patients
who have renal insufficiency secondary to BPH, refractory urinary
retention secondary to BPH, recurrent urinary tract infections,
recurrent bladder stones or gross hematuria due to BPH, and/
or LUTS attributed to BPH refractory to and/or unwilling to use
other therapies.*

We agree with the guidelines that in the management of bothersome
LUTS, it's important that providers recognize the complex dynamics of
the bladder, bladder neck, prostate, and urethra, in addition to the fact
that symptoms may result from interactions of these organs, as well as
with the central nervous system or other systemic diseases.

Based on the functional complexity of the lower urinary tract, we
believe that the history, physical, and basic assessment is not sufficient in managing many male LUTS patients, especially those considering surgery. We recommend urodynamics to help define the lower
urinary tract dysfunction and to individualize the best diagnosis to
treatment pathway.

This module will concentrate on a number of types of male patients
with lower urinary tract symptoms that are commonly seen in clinical
practice. Our hope is to provide you with a real world experience that
shines the light on the benefit of urodynamics in this population.

CASE 1

Elderly Male with Urinary Retention

Diagnosis

History

David is a 83-year-old male with urinary retention. Unable to void, he was recently catheterized for 1200 mL. He was started on an alpha-adrenergic antagonist and treated for constipation.

Prior he was voiding every 1–2 hours with a slow flow. He was getting up three times during the night to urinate.

He has failed two voiding trials and was referred for management.

He has no history of urinary tract infections, previous genitourinary surgery, or risk factors for neurogenic bladder. He has multiple medical comorbidities and is on a number of medications.

David is an elderly male with urinary retention, and has failed two voiding trials on alpha-blockers. He has chronic LUTS secondary to BPH and multiple medical comorbidities. He was evaluated with cystoscopy and urodynamics.

Physical exam

On examination, he has a 50-gram prostate and normal male genitalia. Foley catheter is draining clear urine.

Urinalysis

WBC's and rare bacteria, urine culture negative

Cystoscopy

Patient had bilobar enlargement of prostate and a normal urethra. He had moderate bladder trabeculation and no other intravesical abnormalities.

Urodynamics

David (A)

During urodynamics, the patient had a MCC of 624 mL associated with normal bladder sensation. He had no detrusor overactivity and compliance was normal. He had no urodynamic SUI. During pressure flow his P_{det}max was 82 cmH$_2$O and Qmax was 7 mL/sec. The contraction was

Figure M6-1: David (A) urodynamics

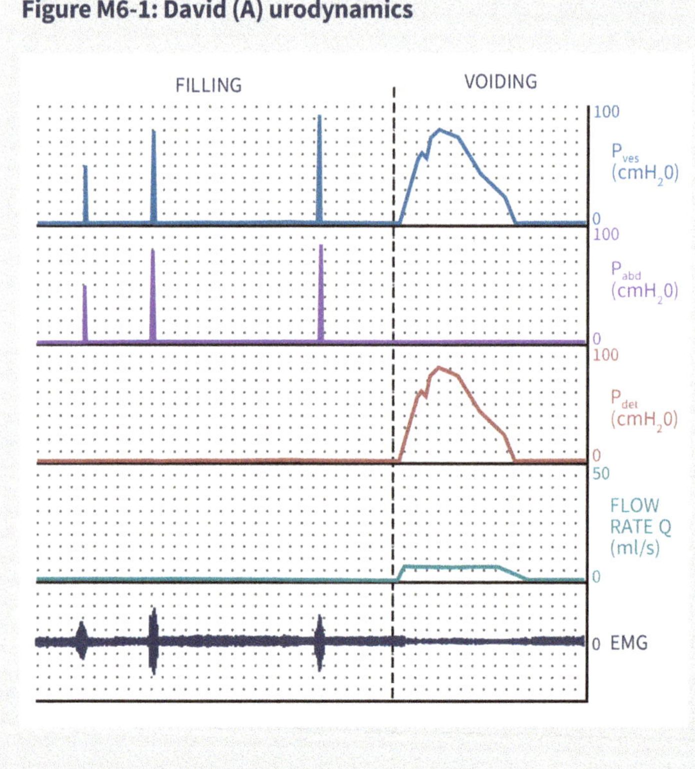

well sustained, and he voided a moderate amount. EMG activity was normal and the PVR was 400 mL (Figure M6-1).

David (B)

During urodynamics, the patient had a MCC of 612 mL associated with normal bladder sensation. He had low pressure detrusor overactivity and compliance was normal. He had no urodynamic SUI. During pressure flow his P_{det}max was 78 cmH_2O and the Qmax was 4 mL/sec. The contraction was poorly sustained, only voiding a small amount. EMG activity was normal and the PVR was 572 mL (Figure M6-2).

Figure M6-2: David (B) urodynamics

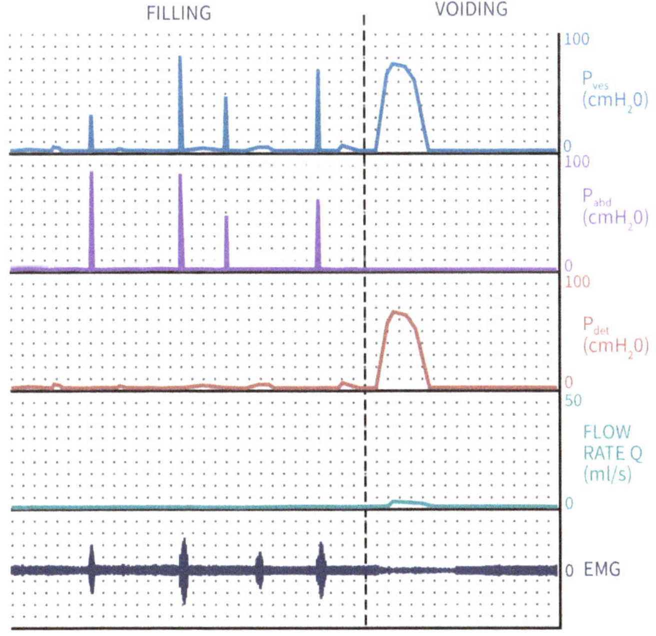

David (C)

During urodynamics, the patient had a MCC of 910 mL associated with decreased bladder sensation. He had low pressure detrusor overactivity and compliance was normal. He had no urodynamic SUI. During pressure flow, his P_{det}max was 28 cmH$_2$O and the Qmax was 9 mL/sec. The contraction was well sustained, and the flow pattern was depressed. EMG activity was normal and the PVR was 731 mL (Figure M6-3).

Figure M6-3: David (C) urodynamics

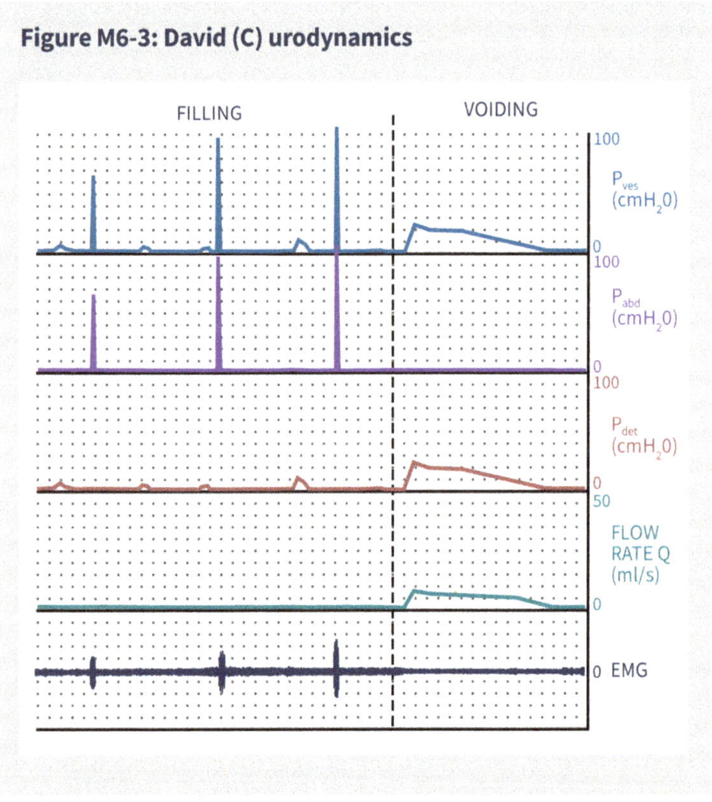

David (D)

During urodynamics, the patient had a MCC of 1200 mL associated with no bladder sensation. Filling cystometry was stopped based on bladder volume. He had no detrusor overactivity and compliance was normal. He had no urodynamic SUI. During pressure flow, he could not generate a voluntary detrusor contraction and failed to void by abdominal straining. EMG activity increased with Valsalva (Figure M6-4).

Figure M6-4: David (D) urodynamics

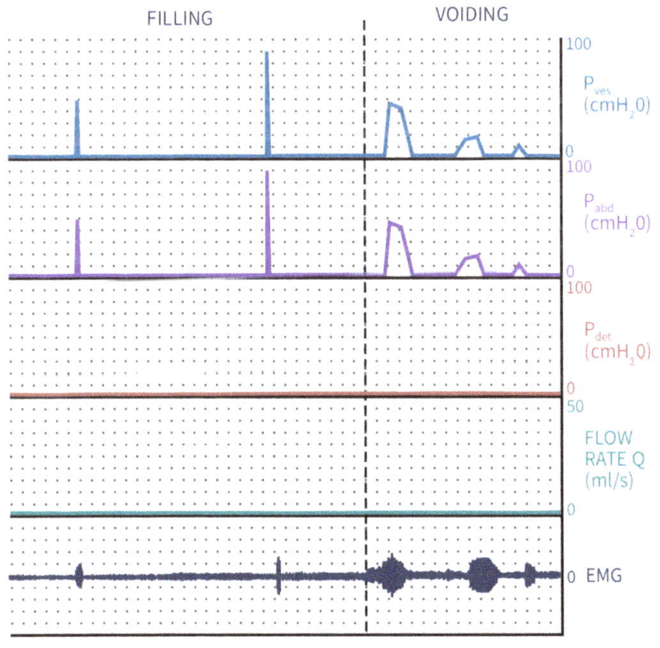

Diagnosis

David (A–D) have urinary retention and chronic LUTS secondary to BPH. They have failed two voiding trials on alpha-blockers.

David (A)

David (A) has normal bladder capacity and favorable bladder storage characteristics. He generates a well sustained high pressure detrusor contraction voiding a small amount. His retention is due to bladder outlet obstruction.

David (B)

David (B) has normal capacity bladder and favorable bladder storage characteristics. He generates a high pressure detrusor contraction that is poorly sustained. His retention is from bladder outlet obstruction, and his poorly sustained detrusor contraction is an aggravating factor.

David (C)

David (C) has a large capacity bladder with decreased bladder sensation and low pressure detrusor overactivity. He generates a normal pressure detrusor contraction that is well sustained. Under normal circumstances, he should be able to empty efficiently. His incomplete emptying is primarily due to bladder outlet obstruction.

David (D)

David (D) has a large capacity bladder associated with no bladder sensation. He is not able to generate a voluntary detrusor contraction even at high volume. His retention is secondary to an acontractile bladder.

Diagnosis to treatment pathway

David (A–D) have urinary retention and chronic LUTS secondary to BPH. They have failed voiding trials on alpha-adrenergic antagonists. Their urodynamic findings influence their individual diagnosis to treatment pathway.

Prostatectomy is successful in treating urinary retention in approximately 90% of cases. Some of the newer minimally invasive procedures appear to be similarly effective. But the efficacy of most surgeries have not been evaluated based on urodynamic findings, which we believe could affect treatment selection and outcome.

A prostatectomy is not a benign procedure and has associated risks, especially in the elderly and those with comorbidities. It's important for patients to have appropriate expectations when consenting for surgery. Lumping all David's into the same "retention group" and counseling and treating them identically is not recommended.

David (A)

- David (A) clearly has high pressure low flow bladder outlet obstruction with no significant filling abnormality. As an "index obstructed patient," he has an excellent surgical prognosis and we would council him accordingly.

David (B)

- David (B) also generates a high pressure detrusor contraction, but it is fleeting in nature. We would recommend surgery, but caution that his success rate is likely lower than an index patient like David (A). A fleeting contraction does not empty as well as one that is well sustained, even if the voiding pressures are similar.

David (C)

- We would similarly lower the surgical success rate in David (C). His large capacity bladder generates a reasonable contraction, but it may not empty well following relief of his obstruction. It's impossible to know if David (C) once had higher pressure voiding and now his contractile strength is beginning to diminish. If David (C)'s normal pressure contraction had been fleeting and poorly sustained his surgical success rate would be even lower.

  If David (B) and (C) become catheter free after surgery they may still have elevated residuals. If their residual remains too high some patients perform CIC once or twice daily to augment voiding. When anticipated, these outcomes are easier to accept and to troubleshoot.

David (D)

- David (D) has a large capacity acontractile bladder and will not be offered surgery. He is an elderly male with medical comorbidities and his surgical success rate is likely less than 10%. Clean intermittent catheterization, a suprapubic tube, and urethral catheter are treatment options. Those recommending a prostatectomy may consider placing a suprapubic tube simultaneously. In a well-informed patient, this is a reasonable strategy.

CASE 2

Middle-Aged Male with Urinary Flow Symptoms

Diagnosis

History

Chris is a 52-year-old male with a poor flow and urinary hesitancy. His stream stops and starts, and he sometimes strains to void. His symptoms have worsened over a decade.

He voids every 1–2 hours and gets up twice during the night to urinate. He has failed an alpha-blocker.

His flow symptoms are significantly impacting his quality of life. He had a lumbar fusion in his early forties secondary to a sports injury. He is otherwise healthy and has no medical comorbidities.

Chris has significant flow symptoms with mild frequency and nocturia. The symptoms are worsening, and he has failed an alpha-blocker. He was evaluated with cystoscopy and urodynamics.

Physical exam

On examination, he has a 40-gram benign prostate and normal male genitalia. He appeared nervous during the evaluation.

Urinalysis

Normal

Postvoid residual

4 mL

Cystoscopy

Patient had a normal urethra with no stricture. He had mild bilobar enlargement of the prostate and an elevated bladder neck. He had impressive bladder trabeculation with a few cellules.

Urodynamics (Video)

Chris (A)

During urodynamics, the patient had an MCC of 524 mL associated with normal bladder sensation. He had no detrusor overactivity and compliance was normal. He had no urodynamic SUI. During pressure flow, his P_{det}max was 66 cmH$_2$O and Qmax was 5 mL/sec. Fluoroscopically, the bladder neck opened immediately, and there was no obstruction at the level of the rhadosphincter. The contraction was well sustained, and he emptied efficiently. EMG activity was normal.

Chris (B)

During urodynamics, the patient had an MCC of 444 mL associated with increased bladder sensation. He had no detrusor overactivity and compliance was normal. He had no urodynamic SUI. He had difficulty voiding in the lab setting, and running water and other provocative maneuvers were utilized. He initially generated a detrusor contraction of 20 cmH$_2$O associated with no flow. Fluoroscopically, he was obstructed at the level of the bladder neck. He finally voided with a P_{det}max of 84 cmH$_2$O and a Qmax of 4 mL/sec. EMG activity was normal.

Figure M6-5: Chris (B) urodynamics

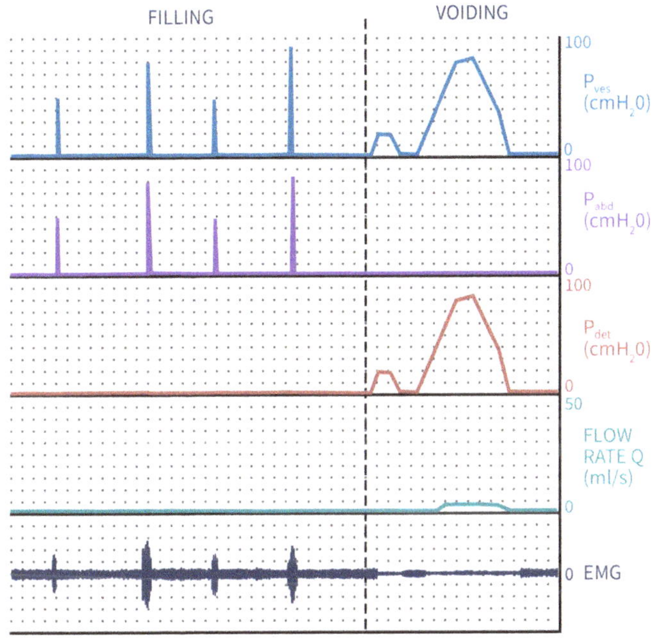

Chris (C)

During urodynamics, the patient had an MCC of 212 mL associated with increased bladder sensation. Bladder filling was limited due to suprapubic pain and pressure and discomfort in the penis. He had low pressure detrusor overactivity and compliance was normal. He had no urodynamic SUI. He had difficulty voiding in the lab setting, and provocative maneuvers were utilized. He voided with a P_{det}max of 61 cmH$_2$O and a Qmax of 9 mL/sec. On fluoroscopy, he was obstructed at the level of rhabdosphincter. EMG activity increased during voiding.

Chris (D)

During urodynamics, the patient had an MCC of 480 mL associated with increased bladder sensation. He had no detrusor overactivity. He had decreased bladder compliance with an end filling pressure of 38 cmH$_2$O. He had no urodynamic SUI. During voiding, he could not generate a detrusor contraction, and emptied by straining. His flow pattern was intermittent with a Qmax of 12 mL/sec. EMG activity increased with Valsalva. He had a Christmas tree-shaped bladder with bilateral grade 2 vesicoureteral reflux.

Chris (E)

During urodynamics, the patient had an MCC of 310 mL associated with increased bladder sensation. He had high pressure detrusor overactivity reaching a pressure of 52 cmH$_2$O. Bladder compliance was normal. He had no urodynamic SUI. He voided with a P$_{det}$max of 20 cmH$_2$O and a Qmax of 18 mL/sec. He reported that his flow and the amount voided was better than usual. EMG activity was normal.

Diagnosis

Chris (A–E) have significant flow symptoms with urinary frequency and nocturia. Their symptoms are worsening and refractory to alpha-adrenergic antagonists.

Chris (A)

Chris (A) has normal bladder capacity with favorable bladder storage characteristics. He is urodynamically obstructed secondary to BPH.

Chris (B)

Chris (B) has normal bladder capacity with favorable bladder storage characteristics. He is urodynamically obstructed at the level of the bladder neck.

Video-urodynamics is necessary to make the diagnosis of bladder neck dyssynergia. Having difficulty voiding in the lab setting is common in this population. Many men with bladder neck dyssynergia are anxious and have a high riding bladder neck cystoscopically.

Chris (C)

Chris (C) has a small capacity bladder limited by pressure and discomfort. He is urodynamically obstructed at the level of the rhabdosphincter. The findings suggest a diagnosis of interstitial cystitis or prostatitis with pelvic floor dyssynergia. Many patients with pelvic floor dyssynergia have difficulty voiding in public settings.

On further questioning, we find that Chris (C) voids frequently due to lower abdominal pressure and less so due to urgency. Sometimes he has mild burning at the tip of the penis during urination. The discomfort may also occur after ejaculation.

Chris (D)

Chris (D) has a normal capacity bladder with increased bladder sensation and loss of bladder compliance. He can't generate a voluntary detrusor contraction and empties by abdominal straining. His significant fluoroscopic findings support a diagnosis of neurogenic bladder dysfunction.

In retrospect, Chris (D) was in retention requiring a catheter for three weeks following his injury and lumbar surgery. He had perineal numbness and difficulty eliminating stool that normalized over time.

Chris (E)

Chris (E) has a small capacity bladder with high pressure detrusor overactivity. His voiding is normal with no evidence of obstruction.

Upon further questioning, Chris (E) describes frequent small volume voiding often associated with urgency. His flow is better first void in the morning and whenever his bladder is full. He voided frequently as a teenager and has always had a "small bladder."

Diagnosis to treatment pathway

Chris (A–E) have worsening flow symptoms with urinary frequency and nocturia. They failed alpha-adrenergic antagonists and are seeking treatment. Their urodynamics influence their individual diagnosis to treatment pathway.

Chris (A)

- Chris (A) has bladder outlet obstruction secondary to BPH and will be recommended prostate surgery. He has an excellent prognosis and we would counsel him accordingly. Some of the minimally invasive procedures that preserve antegrade ejaculation may be preferred.

Chris (B)

- Chris (B) has bladder neck dyssynergia, which is more challenging to treat. Bladder neck incision is the gold standard but usually causes retrograde ejaculation. The rate of ejaculatory dysfunction is lower with unilateral incision, which has been shown to be effective.

Injection of onabotuliumtoxinA into the bladder neck is an off-label treatment option for bladder neck dyssynergia, but its retreatment rate limits its use. A positive response helps confirm the diagnosis, and it's sometimes used for this purpose.

Chris (C)

Chris (C) likely has interstitial cystitis or prostatitis, which can be difficult to differentiate in men.

- We would recommend a bladder hydrodistension for both diagnostic and therapeutic reasons. The presence of glomerulations would establish an IC diagnosis and influence the patient's treatment path. Empiric therapy for IC and prostatitis is also reasonable.

- Chris (C) has high pressure voiding due to pelvic floor dyssynergia. Physical therapy is the treatment of choice for his bothersome flow symptoms and prostate surgery should be avoided.

Chris (D)

- Chris (D) has a neurogenic bladder and strains to urinate. He may wish to perform clean intermittent catheterization instead. It's unlikely that sacral neuromodulation would be efficacious, but a peripheral nerve evaluation is reasonable.
- His neurogenic bladder has not been completely defined, and it's impossible to know the function of his rhadosphincter. Prostate surgery is contraindicated and could result in urinary incontinence, especially if Chris (D)'s distal sphincter has been neurologically compromised.
- Chris (D) should have a renal ultrasound to assess his upper tracts and followed long-term. It is reasonable to ask for a second neurologic opinion from his previous back surgeon.

Chris (E)

- The OAB diagnosis to treatment pathway will be recommended to Chris (E). His poor flow is secondary to small volume voiding, and may improve by increasing his functional capacity with behavioral therapy and OAB agents.
- Third-line treatments can be beneficial, and we would recommend PTNS or sacral neuromodulation. Based on his slow flow, onabotulinumtoxinA may be less ideal. In the absence of having bladder outlet obstruction, we would not recommend prostate surgery to a younger male with voiding dysfunction.

CASE 3

Elderly Male with Lower Urinary Tract Symptoms

Diagnosis

History

Seth is a 73-year-old male with lower urinary tract symptoms. He is bothered by slow flow and urinary hesitancy.

He voids every 30 to 60 minutes and gets up twice during the night to urinate. He has urgency and sometimes experiences urgency incontinence.

He has failed an alpha-adrenergic antagonist and 5-alpha-reductase inhibitor. He is active and has minimal medical comorbidities.

Seth has a slow flow as well as urinary urgency and frequency. He sometimes has urgency incontinence. Since he failed medical therapy he was evaluated with cystoscopy and urodynamics.

Physical exam

On examination, he has a 50-gram benign prostate and normal male genitalia.

Urinalysis

Normal

Postvoid residual

27 mL

Cystoscopy

Patient had a normal urethra and moderate bilobar enlargement of the prostate. He had mild bladder trabeculation and no other abnormalities.

Urodynamics

Seth (A)

During urodynamics, the patient had an MCC of 534 mL associated with normal bladder sensation. He had detrusor overactivity reaching a pressure 6 cmH$_2$O associated with no incontinence. Bladder compliance was normal, and he had no urodynamic SUI. During pressure flow, his P$_{det}$max was 69 cmH$_2$O and Qmax was 4 mL/sec. The contraction was well sustained, and he emptied efficiently. EMG activity was normal.

Seth (B)

During urodynamics, the patient had an MCC of 220 mL associated with increased bladder sensation. He had detrusor overactivity reaching a pressure of 28 cmH$_2$O associated with mild urgency incontinence. Bladder compliance was decreased with an end filling pressure of 29 cmH$_2$O. He had no urodynamic SUI. During pressure flow, his P$_{det}$max was 72 cmH$_2$O and Qmax was 6 mL/sec. The contraction was well sustained, and he emptied efficiently. EMG activity was normal. Fluoroscopically, he had a heavily trabeculated bladder with several diverticula.

Seth (C)

During urodynamics, the patient had an MCC of 357 mL associated with increased bladder sensation. He had detrusor overactivity reaching a pressure of 58 cmH$_2$O associated with high volume urgency incontinence. Bladder compliance was normal, and he had no urodynamic SUI. During pressure flow his P$_{det}$max was 12 cmH$_2$O and Qmax was 6 mL/sec. EMG activity was normal.

Diagnosis

Seth (A–C) have a slow flow and an overactive bladder. They have frequency and intermittent urgency incontinence. They have failed BPH medications.

Seth (A)

Seth (A) has normal bladder capacity with favorable bladder storage characteristics. He is urodynamically obstructed secondary to BPH.

Seth (B)

Seth (B) has decreased bladder capacity with unfavorable bladder storage characteristics. He is urodynamically obstructed secondary to BPH.

Seth (C)

Seth (C) has decreased bladder capacity with unfavorable bladder storage characteristics. His voiding pressure is low, and he is not obstructed.

Diagnosis to treatment pathway

Seth (A–C) have poor flow, frequency, and infrequent urgency incontinence refractory to BPH medication. Their urodynamics influence their individual diagnosis to treatment pathway.

Prostate surgery is an excellent treatment option for male voiding and storage symptoms, especially in those who have bladder outlet obstruction. In the "index" patient, relieving the obstruction generally benefits flow symptoms in approximately 90% of cases. Storage symptoms improve in about 65%, persist in a third, and worsen in 1–2%. Some of the newer minimally invasive procedures appear to provide similar efficacy.

Seth (A)

- We would recommend Seth (A) prostate surgery using the index template. He has normal bladder capacity and favorable bladder storage characteristics. His overactive bladder may take months to improve, and any persisting symptoms could be managed with the OAB diagnosis to treatment pathway.

Seth (B)

- We would be more cautious offering Seth (B) prostate surgery, and would modify our index patient discussion. He has unfavorable bladder storage characteristics, and his OAB is more likely to persist postoperatively. His poor bladder compliance and fluoroscopic findings are chronic changes that place him at higher risk of persistent or worsening symptoms.

Seth (C)

- Seth (C) will be managed using the OAB diagnosis to treatment pathway and not prostate surgery. He is not obstructed, and his unfavorable bladder storage characteristics are likely to persist. Removing his proximal urethral sphincter could cause worsening urgency incontinence secondary to his high pressure detrusor overactivity.

Patient goals and expectations have an impact on treatment. Those who can live with their slow flow can be symptomatically managed with the OAB diagnosis to treatment pathway. The risk of retention with OAB agents as monotherapy or in combination is probably higher in obstructed patients, but the incidence is low even in those with elevated residuals. Their PVR should be followed long-term.

Sacral neuromodulation and PTNS are treatment options for Seth (A–C)'s overactive bladder. Urinary retention rates with onabotulinumtoxinA may be higher in Seth (A) and (B) who have bladder outlet obstruction.

Managing OAB in men and accepting their bladder outlet obstruction is a sound treatment strategy. The natural history of obstruction in not predictable in an individual patient, and we need to be careful using it to justify therapy. The vast majority of symptomatic men with a Qmax < 10 ml/sec are urodynamically obstructed and, for, decades, have been successfully managed with watchful waiting, medication, and various minimally invasive procedures, none of which lower voiding pressure. Until recently, only prostatectomy successfully reduced voiding pressures by eliminating the obstruction.

Male Overactive Bladder Syndrome: Diagnosis to Treatment Pathway

Overactive bladder affects millions of men who are commonly seen in clinical practice. The syndrome is defined as urinary urgency, usually accompanied by urinary frequency and nocturia, with or without urgency urinary incontinence, in the absence of a UTI or other obvious pathology.

Who has OAB versus BPH/BPO is a frequently asked question. The BPH/BPO lower urinary tract storage symptoms are OAB symptoms. The difference between the two diagnoses is terminology and not clinical – although there is discussion about the pathophysiology of idiopathic OAB and storage symptoms secondary to the obstruction. Therefore, it is essentially the same patient with OAB in both cases. In contrast, men who primarily have voiding symptoms without urinary urgency and frequency are coined LUTS secondary to BPH/BPO and primarily have outflow symptoms only.

OAB is defined as being idiopathic, but it's important to look for underlying causes. These may be classified as intravesical, neurologic, or obstructive. The majority of our OAB discussion has been detailed elsewhere and will not be repeated. This module will concentrate on the use of urodynamics in men with OAB who are refractory to conservative therapy.

CASE 1

Male Patient with Overactive Bladder

Diagnosis

History

Sam is a 67-year-old male with a two-year history of urgency, frequency, and nocturia. He voids every 30–60 minutes and twice during the night. He can't sit through a two-hour movie and rushes to the restroom because of urgency. He has no urinary incontinence.

His flow is good, especially first thing in the AM. He has no hesitancy and feels empty after urination.

Sam's symptoms are significantly impacting his quality of life. He has minimal medical comorbidities.

Sam has urinary urgency, frequency, and mild nocturia. He has an overactive bladder and no associated voiding symptoms. He was initially evaluated with a basic assessment, but later with cystoscopy and urodynamics when his symptoms became refractory to treatment.

Physical exam

On examination, the patient has normal genitalia and a 50-gram benign feeling prostate.

Post-void residual urine volume

16 mL

Urinalysis

Normal

Cystoscopy

The patient had mild to moderate bilobar enlargement of the prostate and a normal urethra. He had mild bladder trabeculation but otherwise a normal bladder.

Urodynamics

Sam (A)

During urodynamics, the patient had a MCC of 230 mL associated with increased bladder sensation. He had repetitive high pressure detrusor overactivity reaching a pressure of 59 cmH$_2$O. He had urgency and leaked a few drops. He had no urodynamic SUI. During pressure flow, his P$_{det}$max was 22 cmH$_2$O and the Qmax was 18 mL/sec. The flow pattern and EMG activity were normal (Figure M7-1).

Figure M7-1: Sam (A) urodynamics

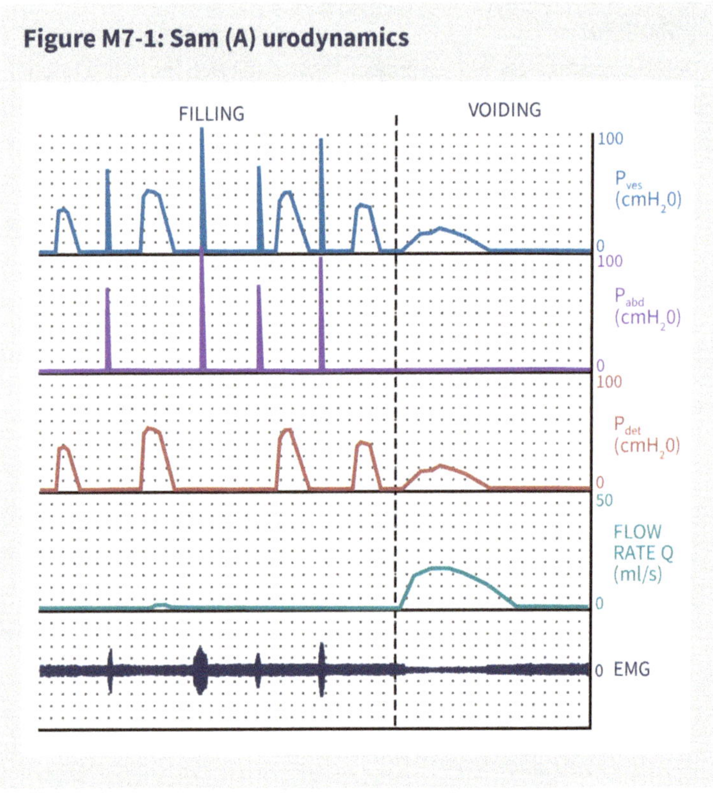

Sam (B)

During urodynamics, the patient had a MCC of 452 mL associated with increased bladder sensation. He had low pressure detrusor overactivity associated with urgency. He had no urodynamic SUI. During pressure flow, his P_{det}max was 26 cmH$_2$O and the Qmax was 16 mL/sec. The flow pattern and EMG activity were normal (Figure M7-2).

Figure M7-2: Sam (B) urodynamics

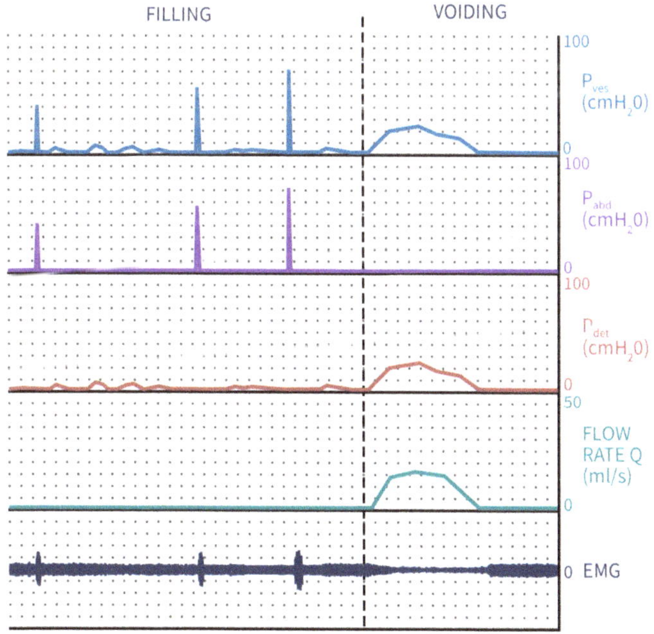

Sam (C)

During urodynamics, the patient had a MCC of 401 mL associated with increased bladder sensation. He had low pressure detrusor overactivity associated with urgency. He had no urodynamic SUI. During pressure flow, his P_{det}max was 78 cmH$_2$O and the Qmax was 20 mL/sec. The flow pattern and EMG activity were normal (Figure M7-3).

Figure M7-3: Sam (C) urodynamics

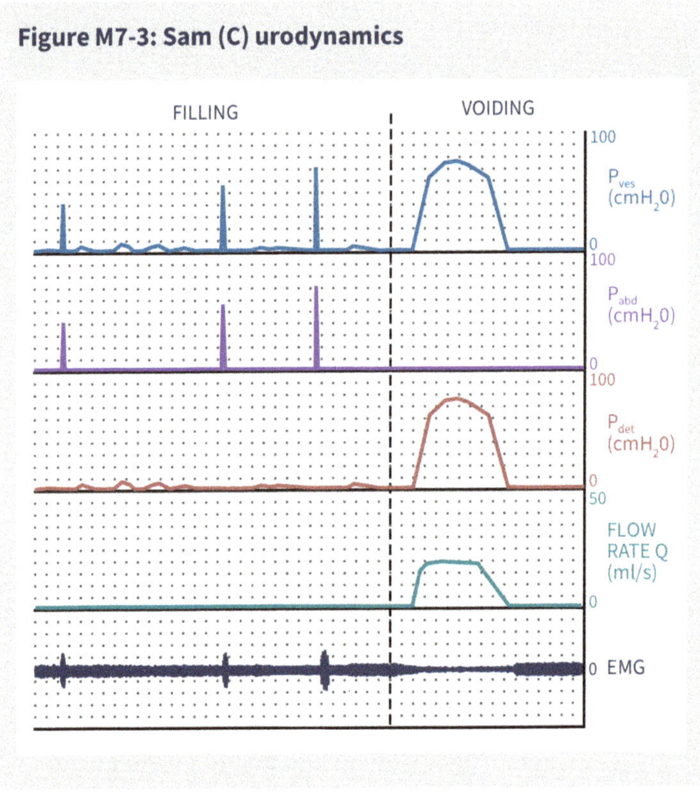

Sam (D)

During urodynamics, the patient had a MCC of 301 mL associated with increased bladder sensation. He had low pressure detrusor overactivity associated with urgency. He had loss of bladder compliance with an end filling pressure of 20 cmH_2O. He had no urodynamic SUI. During pressure flow, his P_{det}max was 62 cmH_2O and the Qmax was 8 mL/sec. The flow pattern was depressed and prolonged. EMG activity was normal (Figure M7-4).

Figure M7-4: Sam (D) urodynamics

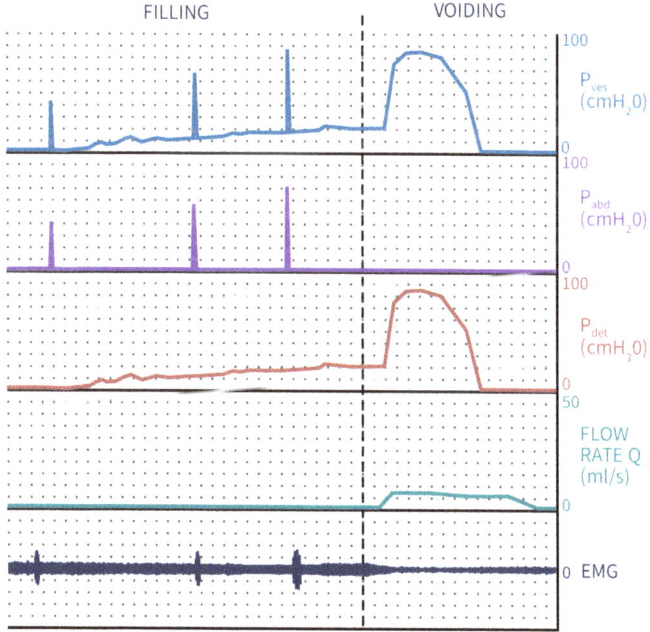

Diagnosis

Sam (A-D) have an overactive bladder affecting their quality of life. They have significant frequency and urgency with mild nocturia. They have no risk factors for voiding dysfunction.

We would initially prescribe an alpha-adrenergic antagonist which can improve storage symptoms. Millions of male LUTS patients report improvement in their OAB symptoms with alpha blockers. Generally speaking, it's a one and done trial, and those who fail can be moved on to other therapies. Otherwise, Sam will be treated with the OAB diagnosis to treatment pathway. Medical and behavioral therapy will be recommended, similar to females. Switch therapy, dose-escalation, and combining OAB agents are effective strategies.

Sam's treatment is more challenging when their symptoms become refractory to medical therapy. Whether they should be treated with the OAB versus the BPH diagnosis to treatment pathway is controversial. Cystoscopy and urodynamics are performed to assess for other pathology and to recommend the best treatment strategy.

Sam (A-D) have urgency and frequency affecting their quality of life. Their symptoms were refractory to alpha-adrenergic antagonists, OAB agents, and behavioral therapy.

Sam (A)

Sam (A) has a small capacity bladder with high pressure detrusor overactivity. He has unfavorable bladder storage characteristics and no bladder outlet obstruction.

Sam (B)

Sam (B) has increased bladder sensation and low pressure detrusor overactivity. He has favorable bladder storage characteristics and no bladder outlet obstruction.

Sam (C)

Sam (C) has increased bladder sensation and low pressure detrusor overactivity. He is urodynamically obstructed with a high voiding pressure and normal flow.

Sam (D)

Sam (D) has a small capacity bladder and increased bladder sensation. He has low pressure detrusor overactivity and loss of compliance. He is urodynamically obstructed with high voiding pressure and low flow.

Diagnosis to treatment pathway

Sam (A–D) have refractory OAB and urodynamics influence their individual diagnosis to treatment pathway.

Sam (A and B)

- Sam (A) and (B) have an overactive detrusor and are not obstructed. They will be treated with third-line OAB therapies including PTNS, onabotulinumtoxinA, and sacral neuromodulation. In the absence of them having flow symptoms or bladder outlet obstruction, we would not offer prostate surgery. For those with a differing viewpoint, prostate procedures may be effective, but success rates are lower in the absence of obstruction. Furthermore, Sam (A)'s unfavorable bladder storage characteristics and its associated symptoms are more likely to persist postoperatively.

Sam (C)

- The management of Sam (C) varies depending on treatment philosophy. He has a high pressure normal flow obstructed bladder and detrusor overactivity. The natural history of obstruction is unpredictable in individual patients, and we need to be careful using it to justify therapy.

- For those willing to accept his bladder outlet obstruction, Sam (C)'s symptoms can be effectively managed with third-line therapies. He may be a higher risk of urinary retention with onabotulinumtoxinA. Prostate procedures to relieve the obstruction are a sound choice. When surgery is effective, it may take 2–4 months for the OAB symptoms to respond. In the absence of having unfavorable bladder storage characteristics, Sam (C)'s prognosis may be more favorable.

Sam (D)

- Sam (D) has loss of bladder compliance secondary to chronic bladder outlet obstruction. Prostate surgery can be offered, but his OAB could persist or worsen due to his poor compliance. Third-line therapies and accepting the obstruction is a reasonable strategy and eliminates this risk. Whether or not refractory OAB treatments are less effective in patients with poor compliance is unknown. Sam should have an upper tract study and be followed long-term for worsening compliance and potential hydronephrosis.

Post-Prostatectomy Incontinence: Diagnosis to Treatment Pathway

Urinary incontinence following radical prostatectomy occurs in approximately 4–8% of cases. The severity varies, as does its impact on quality of life. When incontinence persists for greater than 6–12 months surgery is considered.

The AUA/SUFU guidelines address the management of urinary incontinence after prostate treatment (IPT), including radical prostatectomy (RP), radiation treatment (RT), and treatment of benign prostatic hyperplasia (BPH). Evaluation of IPT and a stepwise approach to its management is discussed.

Guidelines

Clinicians should evaluate patients with incontinence after prostate treatment with history, physical exam, and appropriate diagnostic modalities to categorize type and severity of incontinence and degree of bother.

Prior to surgical intervention for stress urinary incontinence, cystourethroscopy should be performed to assess for urethral and bladder pathology that may affect outcomes or surgery.

Clinicians may perform urodynamic testing in a patient prior to surgical intervention for stress urinary incontinence in cases where it may facilitate diagnosis or counseling.

We agree that cystoscopy evaluates for the presence of a urethral stricture, bladder neck contracture, or bladder pathology that may influence therapy or outcome. Bladder neck calcifications, surgical clips, and radiation changes may also be identified. Placement of an artificial sphincter or male sling necessitates healthy urethral tissue for safe and successful implantation.

The role of urodynamics varies according to patient type and, to some extent, treatment philosophy. While many do not perform urodynamics in men with postprostatectomy incontinence (PPI), we recommend it. We agree with the guidelines that it facilitates diagnosis and hence the individual diagnosis to treatment pathway. It also helps in preoperative counseling and in troubleshooting when necessary.

We will present a number of cases demonstrating the usefulness of urodynamics in this sometimes challenging population of patients.

CASE 1

Index Patient with Urinary Incontinence After Prostatectomy

Diagnosis

History

Gary is a 71-year-old male with urinary incontinence following a robotic assisted radical prostatectomy two years prior. He leaks with coughing, sneezing, bending, and while working in the yard. He wears 4 pads daily to manage his incontinence. Some pads are damp while others are soaked when he is active.

For many years, he has voided every hour, and gets up twice during the night to urinate. He has urgency and has experienced rare urgency incontinence. He has a slow to moderate flow and feels empty after urination.

Gary is right-handed and has not has an abdominal hernia repair. He has minimal medical comorbidities and is seeking treatment for his urinary incontinence.

Gary has post-prostatectomy incontinence that is moderately severe, especially when he is active. He has a long history of having an overactive bladder that has persisted postoperatively. He was evaluated with cystoscopy and urodynamics.

Physical exam

On examination, the patient has normal genitalia and a positive cough test in the standing position. He is not obese, his scrotum is easily palpable, and his hand dexterity is normal. He has no urinary dermatitis or unexpected lower abdominal scars.

Post-void residual urine volume

16 mL

Urinalysis

Normal

Cystoscopy

Absent prostate with coaptation of the membranous urethra. No urethral or bladder pathology identified.

Urodynamics

Gary (A)

During urodynamics, the patient had a MCC of 524 mL associated with normal bladder sensation. He had no detrusor overactivity and compliance was normal. He had urodynamic SUI with a LPP of 90 cmH$_2$O leaking a small amount. Pressure flow and EMG were normal.

Gary (B)

During urodynamics, the patient had a MCC of 524 mL associated with normal bladder sensation. He had no detrusor overactivity and compliance was normal. He had urodynamic SUI with a LPP of 12 cmH$_2$O leaking a large amount. Pressure flow and EMG were normal.

Gary (C)

During urodynamics, the patient had a MCC of 424 mL and mild increased bladder sensation. He had low pressure detrusor overactivity and leaked a few drops. He had mild loss of bladder compliance with an end filling pressure of 16 cmH$_2$O. He had urodynamic SUI with a LPP of 60 cmH$_2$O. Pressure flow and EMG were normal.

Gary (D)

During urodynamics, the patient had a MCC of 244 mL associated with increased bladder sensation. He had repetitive high pressure detrusor overactivity reaching a pressure of 58 cmH$_2$O and associated with high volume urgency incontinence. He was refilled to assess LPP's and voiding. He had urodynamic SUI with a LPP of 60 cmH$_2$O. Pressure flow and EMG were normal.

Gary (E)

During urodynamics, the patient had a MCC of 914 mL associated with decreased bladder sensation. He had detrusor overactivity reaching a pressure of 16 cmH$_2$O and did not leak. He had urodynamic SUI with a LPP of 60 cmH$_2$O. During voiding, he could not generate a detrusor contraction and emptied by Valsalva. EMG activity increased with straining.

Diagnosis

Gary (A–E) have post-prostatectomy incontinence and baseline OAB. Their SUI is moderately severe especially when active.

Gary (A)

Gary (A) has normal bladder filling and emptying and a high leak point pressure. He has favorable bladder storage characteristics and empties efficiently.

Gary (B)

Gary (B) has normal bladder filling and emptying and a significantly low leak point pressure. He has favorable bladder storage characteristics and empties efficiently.

Gary (C)

Gary (C) has normal bladder capacity and low pressure detrusor overactivity leaking a small amount. He has mild loss of bladder compliance. He has a moderately impaired LPP and voids normally.

Gary (D)

Gary (D) has a small capacity bladder with increased bladder sensation. He has impressive high pressure detrusor overactivity, leaking a large amount. He has a moderately impaired LPP and voids normally.

Gary (E)

Gary (E) has a large capacity bladder with decreased bladder sensation. He has low pressure detrusor overactivity and did not leak. He has a moderately impaired LPP and voids by Valsalva.

Diagnosis to treatment pathway

Gary (A–E) have post-prostatectomy incontinence with an overactive bladder. They have flow symptoms but empty efficiently. Based on the history Gary represents the typical or "index" PPI patient commonly seen in clinical practice. Urodynamics help in differentiating one Gary from the others, and these findings require modification of their individual diagnosis to treatment pathways.

The guidelines make a number of statements regarding management of incontinence after prostate treatment.

Guidelines

In patients seeking treatment of incontinence after radical prostatectomy, pelvic floor muscle exercises or pelvic floor muscle training should be offered.

Behavioral therapy and pelvic floor muscle training are effective in milder and motivated patients. Some believe the time to maximum improvement is shorter, but the endgame is the same as watchful waiting and allowing for the urethral sphincter to heal and regain its function. Pelvic floor exercises do benefit overactive bladder symptoms. Teaching pelvic floor therapy prior to surgery is well received by patients.

Guidelines

Patients with urgency incontinence or urgency predominant mixed urinary incontinence should be offered treatment options per the American Urological Association Overactive Bladder guideline.

Many men with post-prostatectomy incontinence have an overactive bladder and mixed urinary incontinence. Detrusor overactivity commonly occurs with aging, or it may result from bladder denervation at the time of surgery. During urodynamics, PPI patients often have a small capacity bladder with increased bladder sensation, and many have mild loss of bladder compliance. A bladder neck contracture may be the source of post-operative obstruction.

We initially manage mixed patients with behavioral therapy and OAB agents. It's rewarding reaching a patient's treatment goal with medication and sparing them surgery.

Refractory patients with mixed incontinence generally do well with a male sling or artificial urinary sphincter, but sometimes their OAB can persist postoperatively. Having already identified and treated their overactive bladder, those with persistent UUI are more understanding and easier to troubleshoot.

Guidelines

An artificial urinary sphincter should be considered for patients with bothersome stress urinary incontinence after prostate treatment. Multiple studies have demonstrated its long-term efficacy and high patient satisfaction in men with any level of bothersome SUI.

The male sling should be considered as a treatment option for mild to moderate stress urinary incontinence after prostate treatment. It should not be routinely performed in patients with severe stress incontinence.

The definition of severe SUI is vague and not universally accepted. Many use a daily pad count of five or greater that are moderately wet as tending towards being severe. Soaking eight pads daily and not voiding because of total incontinence is severe PPI and should not be treated with a male sling. The more we push the severity envelope, the more we have realized that the male sling is still effective in moderately severe patients.

Guidelines

Adjustable balloon devices may be offered to patients with mild stress urinary incontinence after prostate treatment. Patients with incontinence after prostate treatment should be counseled that efficacy is lower and cure is rare with urethral bulking agents.

We agree that bulking agents are less effective and generally do not offer them to PPI patients. Adjustable balloon devices appear promising, but experience with them is limited.

Gary (A)

- Gary (A) will be offered a male sling and artificial sphincter to treat his stress incontinence. A trial with an OAB agent is reasonable, but his problem is primarily stress related. Physical therapy is a good non-surgical approach.

Gary (B)

- Gary (B) will be treated similarly, but his low leak point pressure should be taken into consideration when recommending a male sling. Although LPP is not an established criteria for defining severity of male PPI, its low value should be considered.

  On further questioning, Gary (B)'s incontinence may have initially been underestimated. When he is active and working in the yard his thick pads are heavily soaked. The male sling is still an option, but its efficacy may be compromised due to his baseline intrinsic sphincter deficiency.

Gary (C)

- Gary (C) will be initially treated with OAB agents and behavioral therapy. He has low pressure detrusor overactivity and mild loss of bladder compliance. A small subset of these patients do well with non-surgical treatment.

  If refractory, Gary (C) will be offered a male sling or artificial sphincter. Even with his cystometric finding, he has a good prognosis, but is at increased risk of persistent OAB postoperatively.

Gary (D)

- Gary (D) has impressive high pressure detrusor overactivity and reduced bladder capacity. He will be treated with medical and behavioral therapy before recommending surgery. Both the male sling and artificial sphincter are options, but his overactive detrusor is likely to persist. Increased functional capacity as a result of the surgery could rarely unmask worsening urgency incontinence. For those with persistent symptoms, OAB agents previously unsuccessful may be effective postoperatively. Knowledege of Gary (D)'s overactive bladder will make troubleshooting easier if he remains symptomatic following surgery.

It's unknown whether Gary (C)'s and (D)'s unfavorable bladder storage characteristics could be adversely affected by a potentially obstructing sling placed near the bladder neck, but the possibility of it doing so should be mentioned. There is evidence in patients with neurogenic bladder that bladder compliance may worsen following implantation of an artificial sphincter. The surgically induced detrusor LPP of 60–70 cmH$_2$O may increase bladder pressure and threaten the upper tracts. This has been less of a concern in non-neurogenic men with post-prostatectomy incontinence.

Gary (E)

- Gary (E) has a large capacity bladder with low pressure detrusor overactivity. During voiding, he could not generate a detrusor contraction and emptied by Valsalva. A trial with an OAB agent is reasonable, but is less likely to be effective. An artificial sphincter is a good treatment choice, since it will not obstruct flow or impair emptying. Whether or not the male sling is more likely to cause urinary retention or long-term urinary flow symptoms in this population is unknown. The urodynamic findings are not a contraindication to a sling, but should be taken into consideration and discussed with the patient.

CASE 2

Patient with Worsening Urinary Incontinence Years Following a Prostatectomy

Diagnosis

History

Jim is a 74-year-old male with a seven month history of worsening urinary incontinence. He had a robotic assisted radical prostatectomy nine years prior. Soon after surgery he had salvage external beam radiation, and his most recent PSA is undetectable.

Following his prostatectomy, he leaked with coughing and bending and used one light pad per day to manage his incontinence. He now reports high volume leakage not associated with awareness, soaking three pads daily. He has urgency but no urgency incontinence.

He voids every 1–2 hours and gets up twice during the night to urinate. He has a good flow and feels empty after urination.

Jim is right handed and has not has an abdominal hernia repair. He has diabetes and had a TIA five years ago. He has normal bowel function and is seeking treatment for his urinary incontinence.

Jim has worsening incontinence several years following his prostatectomy and external beam radiation. He leaks without awareness and has stress urinary incontinence. He has mild OAB and medical comorbidities. He was evaluated with cystoscopy and urodynamics.

Physical exam

On examination, the patient has normal genitalia and a mild positive cough test in the standing position. He is not obese, his scrotum is easily palpable, and his hand dexterity is normal. He has no urinary dermatitis or unexpected lower abdominal scars.

Post-void residual urine volume

22 mL

Urinalysis

Normal

Cystoscopy

Absent prostate with coaptation of the membranous urethra. No urethral or bladder pathology identified.

Urodynamics

Jim (A)

During urodynamics, the patient had a MCC of 524 mL associated with normal bladder sensation. He had no detrusor overactivity and compliance was normal. He had urodynamic SUI with a LPP of 32 cmH_2O leaking a large amount. Pressure flow and EMG were normal (Figure M8-1).

Figure M8-1: Jim (A) urodynamics

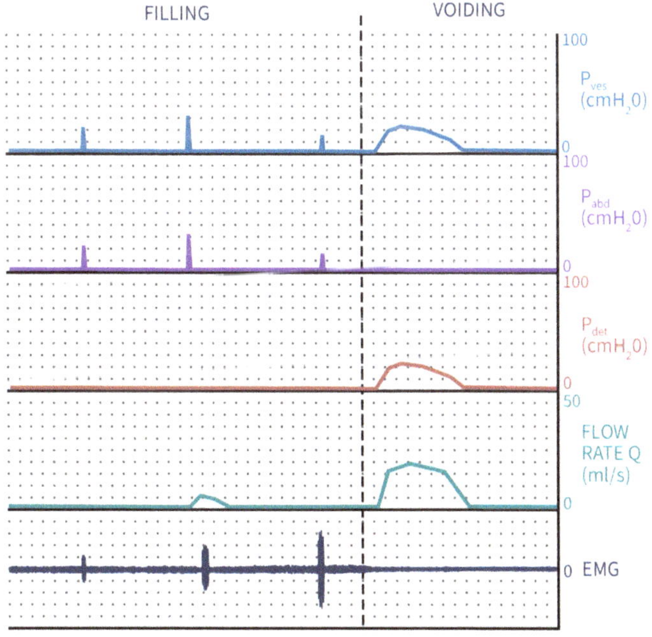

Jim (B)

During urodynamics, the patient had a MCC of 321 mL associated with increased bladder sensation. He had high pressure detrusor overactivity reaching a pressure of 72 cmH_2O and associated with high volume incontinence. He had mild urodynamic SUI with a LPP of 111 cmH_2O. Pressure flow and EMG were normal (Figure M8-2).

Figure M8-2: Jim (B) urodynamics

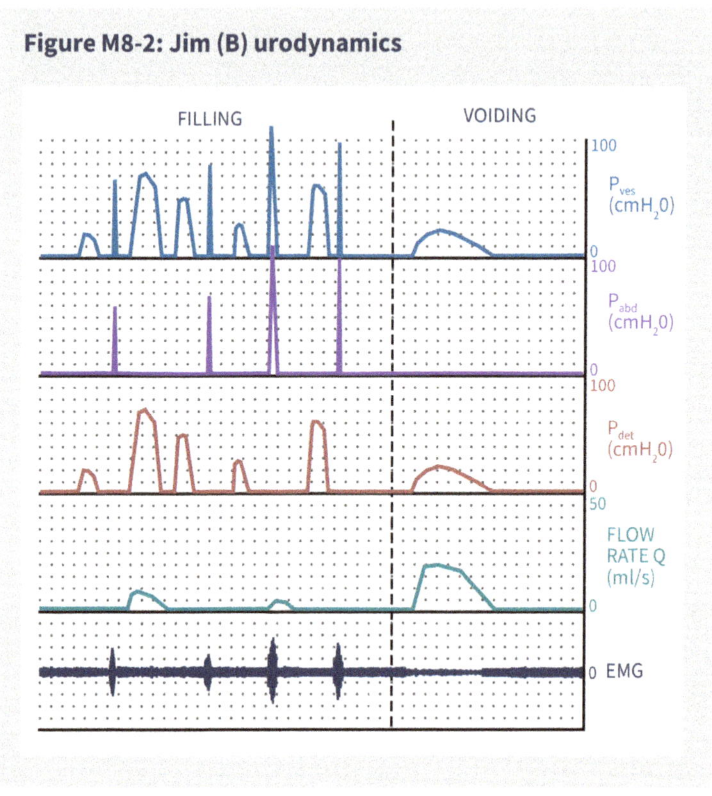

Jim (C)

During urodynamics, the patient had a MCC of 138 mL and increased bladder sensation. He had low pressure detrusor overactivity leaking a few drops. He had loss of bladder compliance with an end filling pressure of 31 cmH$_2$O. He had no urodynamic SUI with the urethral catheter in place, and it had to be later removed to evaluate his stress incontinence. Using the rectal line, his LPP was 128 cmH$_2$O leaking a few drops. Pressure flow and EMG were normal (Figure M8-3).

Figure M8-3: Jim (C) urodynamics

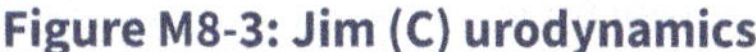

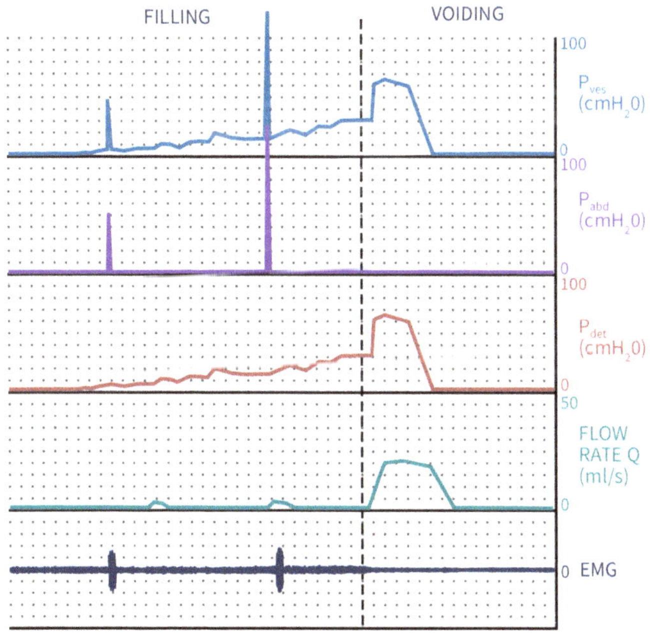

Diagnosis

Jim (A-C) have worsening urinary incontinence years following their prostatectomy and external beam radiation. Initially they had mild stress incontinence, but they now also experience leakage not associated with awareness and urinary urgency. They have additional risk factors for bladder dysfunction.

Radiation can cause a small capacity overactive detrusor with or without loss of compliance. Even in the absence of cystoscopic findings, the effects of radiation commonly present years later, and may worsen over time. Secondary detrusor dysfunction and fibrosis can be refractory to therapy. Radiation can also slowly impact sphincteric function, causing de novo or worsening stress incontinence.

Aging, diabetes, distant stroke, and others are risk factors for developing symptomatic detrusor overactivity and leakage not associated with awareness. Patients who are initially continent or minimally symptomatic after surgery can experience worsening incontinence due to these conditions. Most of these adversely affect the bladder and not the urethral sphincter. Urodynamics are important in differentiating an overactive detrusor from an incompetent outlet.

Jim (A)

Jim (A) has normal bladder filling and emptying and a low leak point pressure. His insensate urine loss is due to urethral incompetence and not an overactive detrusor. Radiation or an aging sphincter may be the underlying cause.

Jim (B)

Jim (B) has reduced bladder capacity and high pressure detrusor overactivity. His high LPP corresponds with his long-term SUI, but not his worsening leakage not associated with awareness. His unfavorable bladder storage characteristics are the cause of his high volume insensate urinary incontinence.

Jim (C)

Jim (C) has a small capacity bladder and low pressure detrusor overactivity. His poor bladder compliance may be secondary to radiation, surgically associated bladder denervation, or previous long-term bladder outlet obstruction. His urodynamic SUI is mild and is not the cause of his leakage without awareness. As is the case with Jim (B), the culprit is his unfavorable bladder.

Diagnosis to treatment pathway

Jim (A–C) have significant leakage not associated with awareness beginning years following their prostatectomy and radiation. They have long-term SUI and risk factors for worsening incontinence. Their urodynamics influence their individual diagnosis to treatment pathway.

Jim (A)

- Jim (A) will be offered an artificial sphincter to treat his stress urinary incontinence.

Guidelines

We agree with the guidelines that men with stress incontinence after primary, adjuvant, or salvage radiotherapy who are seeking surgical management, artificial urinary sphincter is preferred over a male sling or adjustable balloons.

An artificial sphincter is safe and effective in radiated patients. Preoperative cystoscopy usually demonstrates a normal bulbar urethra distant from the radiated field. It has been well established that erosion and infection rates are slightly higher, but the long-term success rate is similar to those who are not radiated. A transcorporal cuff may be considered after pelvic irradiation when indicated.

The male sling is not recommended in radiated patients, and it may not be a good choice if radiation therapy is anticipated. Although radiation is not an absolute contraindication, the fear of erosion has limited its use by the majority of urologists. A mesh erosion into a radiated urethra or bladder neck is serious and difficult to manage. Many patients successfully managed with a male sling develop de novo stress incontinence soon after radiation, likely due to urethral atrophy associated with the therapy.

Jim (B)

- Jim (B) will be offered OAB agents and behavioral therapy to address his leakage not associated with awareness. The OAB diagnosis to treatment pathway including third-line therapies will be used. OnabotulinumtoxinA is not approved in radiated patients, but appears to be safe. His well-tolerated mild SUI will not be treated.

Jim (C)

- Jim (C) will also be treated with first, second, and third-line OAB therapies. For some patients, it's reasonable to perform an examination under anesthesia to measure their true bladder capacity, especially in those considering onabotulinumtoxinA. The first injection could be done simultaneously. A small fibrosed radiated detrusor has a poor prognosis and demands long-term upper tract surveillance. The efficacy of all OAB therapies is lower in this population of patients, and patient expectations should be clarified.

CASE 3

Urinary Incontinence in a Male with an Artificial Urinary Sphincter

Troubleshooting incontinence in patients with an artificial sphincter is best done with a stepwise approach. The device is prone to a number of problems, including urethral atrophy, loss of volume, erosion, and infection. Differentiating between a bladder storage disorder and a malfunctioning device is also important.

The history is the first step in diagnosing the problem. It identifies the type of incontinence that, in some cases, is due to an overactive detrusor. Identifying precipitating factors is recommended.

If the patient reports a soft or empty scrotal pump, it generally means loss of volume. More squeezes required to cycle the device suggests urethral atrophy and subsequent stress incontinence. Each squeeze transfers approximately 0.5 mL of normal saline back to the abdominal reservoir. A normal cuff has in it approximately 1 mL, needing two pumps to empty. Atrophy allows more fluid to enter the cuff requiring additional squeezes to evacuate.

Hematuria, blood at the meatus, dysuria, and the new onset of incontinence suggest cuff erosion. Urinary tract infections are easily diagnosed. Obstructive symptoms and overflow incontinence can occur from a bladder neck contracture. Patients with an infected device may report pain, swelling, erythema, and tenderness in the perineum, scrotum, and, less commonly, the lower abdomen.

On physical examination, patients with PPI may leak in the standing position with coughing or gravity. Even a well-functioning device can leak a small amount. The stress test is repeated with the cuff open for comparison. Cycling the device evaluates it for mechanical failure.

Incisional drainage, erythema, pain, and swelling indicate infection and can occur years after. A tender cuff may be an early sign versus a draining sinus or exposed implant.

Identifying the location of the cuff along the bulbar urethra is important especially when planning re-exploration. A too distally placed cuff predisposes to SUI, especially as the smaller distal urethra atrophies. Pushing on the cuff through the perineum while performing cystoscopy can better establish cuff position relative to perineal and scrotal landmarks. The information allows planning on whether a new cuff can be safely placed more proximally as a salvage procedure. If not, downsizing the current cuff or adding a second one distally are excellent options.

Sometimes a palpable herniated abdominal reservoir can adversely affect its function. Identifying incisions and tubing is important, especially if revision is considered. A copy of the original operating report and knowing the size of initial cuff is valuable.

Urinalysis and culture identify infection and blood in the urine. The absence of microscopic hematuria does not rule out cuff erosion. An elevated post-void residual may be secondary to a bladder neck contracture.

During cystoscopy, the cuff is evaluated both closed and opened. Erosion is easily identified, and the presence of erythema may suggest a pending one. Nighttime deactivation may help salvage a near urethral erosion.

Cuff occlusion should be judged endoscopically. A poorly functioning open cuff is easily visualized, but a smaller opening can be difficult to detect. A closed urethra supports adequate device function, but it does not rule out SUI diagnosed by leak point pressure.

Evaluation of the bladder neck and bladder is important to look for other pathology. Damaging the sphincter during cystoscopy is rare, and keeping the cuff open by re-cycling the device with the cystoscope in place may minimize the risk.

Urodynamics are used to distinguish between an overactive detrusor and incompetent sphincter. The cuff is opened for catheter insertion and then allowed to close down around the catheter. A well-functioning device will provide a leak point pressure of 60–70 cmH$_2$O or greater. A normal value should be rechecked with the catheter removed since in rare cases it can obstruct and falsely elevate the leak point pressure. The rectal line is used for this repeat evaluation. A lower LPP diagnoses sphincteric weakness.

Cystometry may identify increased bladder sensation, detrusor overactivity, and loss of compliance. The voiding phase is performed with the cuff open and has less relevance in this population. We liberally use antibiotics just prior to and for a few days after the study and warn patients of the rare risk of infection and erosion.

The majority of artificial sphincter patients with worsening incontinence have urethral atrophy, loss of device volume, or an overactive detrusor. Atrophy diminishes cuff function and usually takes a few years to develop. Most incontinence due to mild urethral atrophy stabilizes and is managed conservatively.

When surgically indicated, atrophy is treated by down-sizing the cuff, placing it more proximal, or adding a second cuff downstream in tandem.

Loss of device volume below approximately 19 mL greatly reduces cuff pressure. Opening the abdominal incision and measuring total device volume is an important intraoperative diagnostic step. Complete device replacement is recommended for volume loss and also considered for any malfunction when the device is older than 5 years. Pre-operative abdominal ultrasound to assess the size of the reservoir and for fluid loss can also be performed.

Numerous patients develop an overactive detrusor unrelated to the sphincter. They report urgency incontinence, leakage not associated with awareness, and/or enuresis. The normal functioning device is not able to resist the bladder overactivity. The overactive detrusor is treated with the OAB diagnosis to treatment pathway.

Diagnosis

History

Mike is a 77-year-old male with a one year history of urinary incontinence. He has an artificial sphincter placed six years earlier for post-prostatectomy stress incontinence and was initially dry.

He leaks a small amount with coughing and sneezing but primarily has incontinence not associated with awareness. He wears 3 to 4 pads daily that are moderately wet. He has urgency but no urgency incontinence.

He cycles the device and voids with a good flow. He voids every 2 hours and has mild nocturia. He reports no hematuria, cystitis, or precipitating factors.

Mike is motivated to achieve better continence and has minimal medical comorbidities.

Mike has stress incontinence and leakage not associated with awareness after being continent for years with an artificial sphincter. He was evaluated with cystoscopy and urodynamics.

Physical exam

On examination, the patient has normal genitalia and a mild positive cough test in the standing position. The pump is easily palpated in the dependent right hemi-scrotum, and there are no signs of infection. The device cycles normally.

Post-void residual urine volume

2 mL

Urinalysis

Normal

Cystoscopy

The penile and bulbar urethra are normal. The cuff appears to be occluding well, but there may be a dimple size opening. After cycling the device, there is no evidence of erosion. The bladder neck and bladder are normal.

Urodynamics

Mike (A)

During urodynamics, the patient had a MCC of 524 mL associated with normal bladder sensation. He had no detrusor overactivity, and compliance was normal. He had urodynamic SUI with a LPP of 42 cmH$_2$O leaking a moderate amount. Pressure flow and EMG were normal.

Mike (B)

During urodynamics, the patient had a MCC of 282 mL and increased bladder sensation. He had detrusor overactivity reaching a pressure of 42 cmH$_2$O and high volume leakage not associated with awareness. With and without the urethral catheter in place, he leaked a few drops with a LPP of 88 cmH$_2$O. Pressure flow and EMG were normal.

Diagnosis

Mike (A)

Mike (A) and (B) have worsening leakage not associated with awareness and mild stress incontinence. After enjoying years of continence with an artificial sphincter, they are seeking treatment for their de novo symptoms.

Mike (A) has normal bladder capacity with no detrusor overactivity. He has urodynamic SUI with a moderately low LPP. The study demonstrates sphincter malfunction as the underlying etiology. Urethral atrophy and loss of volume are the most common causes.

Mike (B)

Mike (B) has a small capacity bladder and increased bladder sensation. His leakage without awareness is due to detrusor overactivity and not SUI. The sphincter is working well, leaking only a few drops at high pressure.

Diagnosis to treatment pathway

Mike (A) and (B) have an artificial sphincter with leakage without awareness and mild stress incontinence. Urodynamics are important in recommending their individual diagnosis to treatment pathway.

Mike (A)

- Mike (A) will be treated by re-exploration and troubleshooting the device. If the device has lost volume, it will be replaced. The same size cuff and location will be used, and it will be activated almost immediately. Postoperative scrotal swelling or tenderness may delay activation for 1–2 weeks. Cuff atrophy is managed by down-sizing the cuff, placing one more proximal, or adding a second cuff downstream in tandem. The latter two require 6 weeks of healing before activation. Because the sphincter is six years old, an entirely new device will be implanted.

Mike (B)

- Mike (B) will be managed with first, second, and third-line OAB therapies. The need for repeat cystoscopy in the presence of an artificial urinary sphincter may make onabotulinumtoxinA less desirable.

Neurogenic Bladder Dysfunction: Diagnosis to Treatment Pathway

Neurogenic bladder dysfunction encompasses the abnormal changes in function of the bladder and urethra resulting from lesions of their innervation, either within the central nervous system or in the peripheral nerves of the lower urinary tract.

Discrete lesions at various levels usually affect the bladder and urethra in a relatively consistent fashion. They may be classified into supraspinal, suprasacral, and infrasacral, according to the level of the lesion with regard to the pontine micturition center and conus medullaris where a sacral voiding center exists. Supraspinal lesions include all lesions above the level of the brain stem and pons. Suprasacral are spinal cord lesions above the conus. Infrasacral lesions involve the conus or sacral roots, and may be further subdivided into cauda equina lesions (within the spinal canal) and peripheral nerve lesions (outside the spinal canal).

Supraspinal lesions

Patients with diseases of the cerebral cortex, including stroke, dementia, tumor, and Parkinson's, commonly have voiding dysfunction. Central inhibition of the pontine micturition reflex is lost resulting in uncontrolled reflex bladder contractions and neurogenic detrusor overactivity. An intact pons ensures normal coordination between the bladder and urethral sphincter, maintaining low voiding pressure. Patients with supraspinal lesions do not develop poor bladder compliance threatening renal health.

These patients commonly have urinary frequency, nocturia, urgency, and urgency incontinence. When sensory pathways are affected, they report urinary incontinence not associated with awareness. Many have cognitive or functional impairment adversely affecting continence.

Those with supraspinal lesions usually void and empty efficiently. Incomplete emptying is often due to preexisting bladder dysfunction such as an obstructing prostate. Importantly, some supraspinal lesions effect central voiding centers and neurologically impair bladder contractility.

Spinal shock may occur after an acute cerebral event such as stroke, surgery, or severe concussion. Bladder contractility is temporarily impaired, resulting in retention for a few days or weeks. Urinary retention is best managed by an indwelling catheter or CIC, depending on the patient's functional ability and support staff. A trial of voiding is delayed until mental and physical health improve.

Suprasacral lesions

Patients with spinal cord lesions, including those with spinal cord injury, tumor, transverse myelitis, and multiple sclerosis have neurogenic bladder dysfunction. The discussion of suprasacral lesions is usually directed to those with complete or near complete traumatic spinal cord injuries. Much of what is learned from these patients is transferable to those with other cord conditions.

Spinal shock may last a few weeks to several months. Loss of neurologic activity below the injury results in an acontractile detrusor and urinary retention. Patients are initially managed by indwelling or intermittent catheterization.

Recovery from shock is characterized by the gradual "waking up" of the bladder and return of reflex activity. Emerging detrusor overactivity is mediated through the sacral voiding center, which is intact but separated from higher centers. Patients initially continent become incontinent as they start to involuntarily void. The reflex contractions become stronger, allowing for emptying, but sometimes at the cost of higher detrusor pressure.

Patients with suprasacral lesions usually lose the coordinating effect of the pontine micturition center and develop detrusor sphincter dyssynergia (DSD). DSD is the involuntary contraction of the external sphincter during voiding and is pathognomonic for neurogenic bladder.

The bladder contracts against a closed sphincter, resulting in high voiding pressure and inefficient emptying. Patients with suprasacral lesions can also develop high bladder pressure from poor detrusor compliance and/or high pressure detrusor overactivity (Figure M9-1).

Figure M9-1: Loss of compliance and high voiding pressure in neurogenic bladder with detrusor sphincter dyssynergia, also demonstrated fluoroscopically.

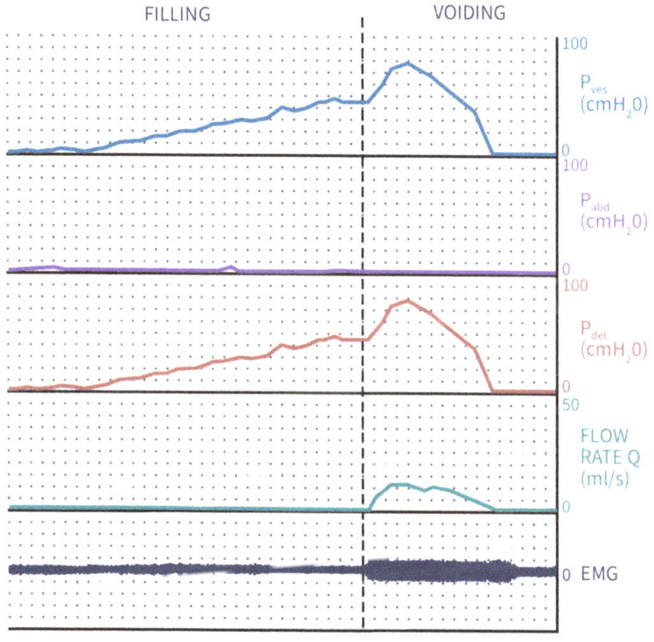

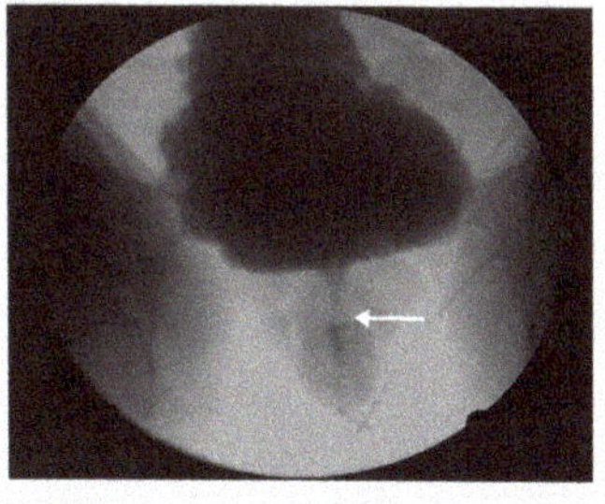

High voiding and filling pressure can lead to both bladder and renal deterioration. It's generally accepted that sustained detrusor pressure > 40 cmH$_2$0 is detrimental to the kidneys. The detrusor muscle thickens and loses its normal sphere, sometimes forming a Christmas tree-shaped bladder with multiple diverticula. Vesicoureteral reflux, hydronephrosis, and renal insufficiency may develop. These silent bladder and renal effects generally take years, but sometimes occur rapidly.

Infrasacral lesions

Infrasacral lesions involve the conus medullaris, the cauda equina, or the peripheral nerves that innervate the bladder and urethra (once termed lower motor neuron lesions). Common causes include spinal cord injury, intervertebral disc disease, and lumbar spinal stenosis. The motor nuclei of the pelvic parasympathetics and pudendal nerves are situated within the conus generally located at the level of the T12 and L1 vertebral bodies. Thoracolumbar sympathetic nuclei also provide fibers that travel in the hypogastric nerves. Injury to the conus and cauda equina may affect bladder function variably, but the dysfunction primarily depends on the extent of injury to the parasympathetic innervation.

Infrasacral lesions most commonly result in an acontractile bladder. The normal reflex arc between the bladder and conus is interrupted. The patient usually presents with obstructive voiding or urinary retention. Many women empty by abdominal straining or by suprapubic pressure. Others develop overflow incontinence or SUI due to a denervated urethral sphincter. Patients commonly have sensory loss in the perineum, perianal area, or lateral aspect of the foot.

Most complete infrasacral patients have large capacity low pressure detrusors. For reasons not fully understood, a significant number of them lose bladder compliance and develop high detrusor pressure. Urodynamics is important in diagnosing this group.

Patients with partial infrasacral lesions behave differently. Partial interruption of the sacral reflex often causes detrusor overactivity. These patients typically preserve voiding but suffer from frequency and urgency incontinence. Partial lesions are commonly seen in patients with lumbar disc disease.

Diagnosis

Millions of patients with neurologic disease suffer from lower urinary tract symptoms. Approximately 1–10% of patients with multiple sclerosis present with voiding dysfunction and urinary incontinence.

Making a diagnosis of neurogenic bladder in those with no known neurologic disease can be challenging. Expert opinion using nonspecific factors, rather than pathognomonic signs and symptoms, is often necessary. An important indicator is a temporal relationship between a potential neurologic event and the patient's symptoms. A clinical presentation out of the ordinary may be the first clue in making the diagnosis. For example, a 36-year-old male who carries a urinal in his car because of urgency and fear of incontinence, or a young healthy woman who begins experiencing flooding bedwetting without an identifiable cause, is not normal.

A thorough history is recommended in patients with neurogenic bladder, and in those suspected of having one. Assessing for the presence of neurologic symptoms is an important aspect of the evaluation. The bowel, bladder, perineum, and lower extremities share sacral cord innervation, which accounts for the associated symptoms. Some patients report loss or decreased sensation in the perineum or genitalia. They may have urgency or insensate urinary or fecal incontinence as well as erectile dysfunction. Others report motor or sensory symptoms involving the lower extremities. The absence of neurologic symptoms does not exclude the diagnosis.

A focused neurologic examination should be performed. The patient's general mental and ambulatory status and lower extremity neuromuscular function is assessed. Positive local findings include sensory loss involving the genitalia and perineum, reduced anal sphincter tone, absent bulbospongiosus reflex, and inability to voluntarily contract the anal sphincter. Palpation and inspection of the lower back and sacrum for dermatologic stigmata of spinal bifida occulta or the presence of sacral agenesis is important.

We recommend urodynamics in nearly all neurogenic patients. Detrusor sphincter dyssynergia is pathognomonic, but only present in select patients. Unfavorable bladder storage characteristics in the appropriate clinical setting suggests the diagnosis. Findings include high pressure detrusor overactivity, loss of bladder compliance, repetitive and similar sinewave detrusor overactivity (Figure M9-2), and sequential overactivity escalating in a stepping pattern, with or without loss of bladder compliance. (Figure M9-3).

Other patients have poor or absent bladder sensation during filling cystometry. Detrusor overactivity that is associated with leakage without awareness is similarly common. Some patients have large capacity poorly contractile detrusors, often with elevated residuals.

Video-urodynamics is preferred since fluoroscopy may reveal cystogram findings suggesting the diagnosis. These include heavy trabeculation, bladder diverticula, a Christmas tree-shaped bladder, vesicoureteral reflux, and detrusor sphincter dyssynergia. DSD can sometimes be more readily visualized radiographically than detected by insensitive patch electrodes.

In spinal cord patients, urodynamics are recommended at 3 and 12 months following the injury. They are generally repeated annually or every alternate year, depending on risk factors for developing high

Figure M9-2: Sine Wave Pattern

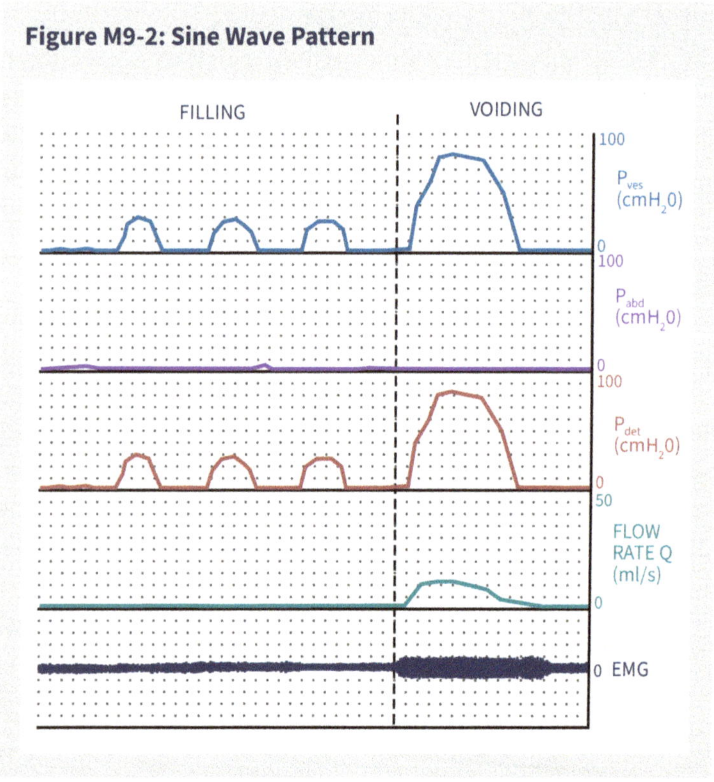

detrusor pressure, or until the patient's bladder dysfunction has stabilized. Other indications for repeating the study include a change in urinary symptoms, hydronephrosis or renal function deterioration, or the new onset of autonomic dysreflexia.

Patients with suprasacral and infrasacral lesions should be followed with a baseline and annual renal ultrasound long-term. When abnormalities are detected, a more diagnostic CT scan may be necessary.

It's important to be aware that some patients with partial suprasacral and infrasacral lesions, and who are minimally symptomatic, can develop high bladder pressure and silently injure their kidneys. This is especially common in men who have competent urethral sphincters. The same high pressure in women usually causes urinary incontinence, protecting their upper tracts. Urodynamics are a necessary pressure test to identify these patients, and empiric symptomatic treatment should be discouraged.

Figure M9-3: Stepping Pattern

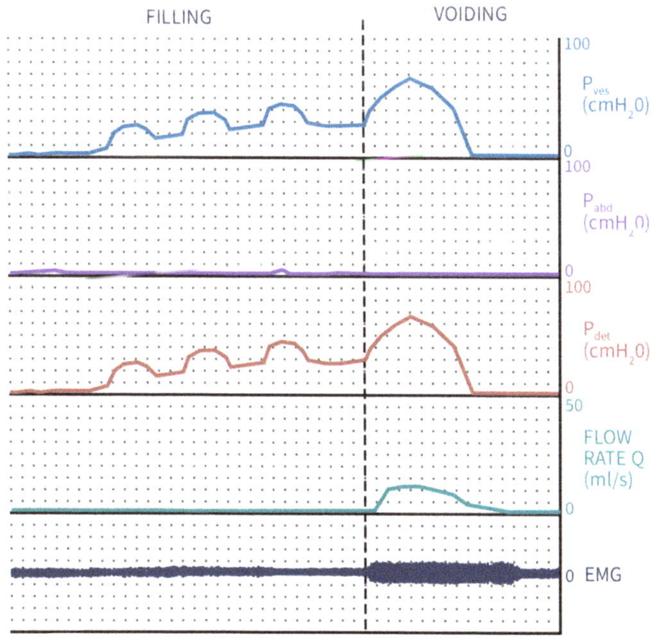

Similarly, many cervical spinal cord patients empty efficiently into a condom catheter, but their voiding pressure may not be safe. Many empty by generating high detrusor pressure secondary to detrusor sphincter dyssynergia, and urodynamics is the only means to identify these patients.

Treatment

Patients with neurogenic bladder are managed with a diagnosis to treatment pathway tailored to the individual. The goals of therapy are to preserve renal function, to achieve adequate bladder emptying and continence, and to minimize urologic complications, including recurrent UTI's and renal calculi. Optimizing patient independence is important.

Symptomatic management of lower urinary tract symptoms is usually effective. Overactive bladder symptoms are treated with behavioral therapy, OAB medication, and refractory third-line treatments. Obstructive symptoms and retention may respond to alpha-adrenergic antagonists.

Surgically treating lower urinary tract symptoms in patients with neurogenic bladder requires careful consideration. A sling in a male or female with SUI has a significant chance of causing retention, while bulking agents or artificial sphincters generally nullify this risk. Obstructive symptoms in men who have absence of bladder contractility or DSD will probably not respond to a transurethral resection of the prostate. Storage symptoms due to neurogenic detrusor overactivity will likely persist or worsen post-prostatectomy or following a bladder neck suspension.

Most patients with urinary retention are treated with clean intermittent catheterization. CIC, in combination with OAB medication, can successfully manage elevated detrusor pressure, urinary incontinence, and reduce UTI's. Many patients with c-spine injury, Parkinson's, or multiple sclerosis lack the necessary hand function to self-catheterize. Others are too obese, immobile, cognitively impaired, or unwilling. It's unrealistic to have caregivers perform CIC, threatening the patient's independence. An indwelling urethral or suprapubic catheter or a urinary diversion may be necessary.

Urinary retention secondary to detrusor sphincter dyssynergia rarely responds to alpha-adrenergic antagonists. CIC is the treatment of choice and very few patients are treated with an irreversible sphincterotomy. OnabotulinumtoxinA injected into the sphincter can be effective, but its durability is limited. Any form of sphincterotomy that improves bladder emptying usually causes urinary incontinence.

OnabotulinumtoxinA is FDA-approved for neurogenic detrusor overactivity. Not only does it improve continence it reduces detrusor pressure. Bladder augmentation is similarly effective but it is less commonly performed since approval of the toxin.

The adult AUA/SUFU urodynamic guidelines address the use of urodynamics in patients with neurogenic bladder.

Guidelines

Clinicians should perform PVR assessment, complex cystometrogram (CMG), pressure flow analysis, and electromyography (EMG) during the initial urological evaluation of patients with relevant neurological conditions with or without symptoms and as part of ongoing follow-up when appropriate, in patients with other neurologic disease and elevated PVR or in patients with LUTS symptoms.

When available, clinicians may perform fluoroscopy at the time of urodynamics (video-urodynamics) in patients with relevant neurologic disease at risk for neurogenic bladder, in patients with other neurologic disease and elevated PVR or in patients with urinary symptoms.

Urodynamics are important in characterizing the vesicourethral dysfunction and detecting elevated detrusor pressure independent of symptoms. In addition, knowledge of how the neurologic disease affects the lower urinary tract and appreciating the impact of any pre-existing dysfunction is essential in recommending the individual diagnosis to treatment pathway. In this module, we will demonstrate the usefulness of urodynamics in this often complex patient population.

CASE 1

Elderly Male with Stroke and Urinary Incontinence

Diagnosis

History

John is a 71-year-old male with urinary incontinence since his stroke 11 months earlier. He has moderately severe urgency incontinence and sometimes leaks without awareness. He uses 4 heavy pads daily that are soaked.

He voids hourly and gets up three times during the night to void. His flow is slow and often associated with urgency. He has terminal straining but feels empty after urination.

He had a poor flow and frequency prior to the stroke but his urinary frequency has worsened.

John has mild right sided weakness and ambulates well with a walker. He has a number of medical comorbidities.

Following a stroke, John has moderately severe urgency incontinence and sometimes leaks without awareness. He has persistent poor flow and his urinary frequency has worsened. Based on the temporal relationship, he was diagnosed as having a neurogenic bladder and was evaluated with urodynamics.

Physical exam

On physical examination, the patient has normal genitalia and a negative cough test in the standing position. He has a 50-gram benign prostate.

Post-void residual

209 mL

Urinalysis

Normal

Urodynamics

John (A)

During urodynamics, the patient had a MCC of 446 mL with mild increased bladder sensation. He had detrusor overactivity reaching pressures of 19 cmH$_2$O associated with mild urgency incontinence. During pressure flow, his P$_{det}$max was 32 cmH$_2$O and the Qmax was 10 mL/sec. The flow pattern was depressed and prolonged. EMG activity was normal and the PVR was 23 mL.

John (B)

During urodynamics, the patient had a MCC of 286 mL with increased bladder sensation. He had detrusor overactivity reaching pressures of 80 cmH$_2$O associated with high volume urgency incontinence. His bladder was refilled to assess voiding. During pressure flow, his P$_{det}$max was 62 cmH$_2$O and the Qmax was 4 mL/sec. The flow pattern was depressed and prolonged. EMG activity was normal and the PVR was 193 mL.

John (C)

During urodynamics, the patient had a MCC of 816 mL with decreased bladder sensation. He had detrusor overactivity reaching pressures of 12 cmH$_2$O and leaked a small amount not associated with awareness. During pressure flow, his P$_{det}$max was 8 cmH$_2$O and the Qmax was 4 mL/sec. The flow pattern was intermittent, and he strained to void. The EMG activity increased with straining and the PVR was 172 mL.

John (D)

During urodynamics, the patient had a MCC of 516 mL with normal bladder sensation. He had significant loss of bladder compliance with an end filling pressure of 31 cmH_2O. He had detrusor overactivity reaching pressures of 12 cmH_2O and did not leak. During pressure flow, his P_{det}max was 50 cmH_2O and the Qmax was 6 mL/sec. The flow pattern was depressed and prolonged. EMG activity was normal and the PVR was 203 mL.

Diagnosis

John (A–D) have urgency incontinence since a stroke and chronic lower urinary tract symptoms secondary to BPH. They have worsening frequency and a functional component to their incontinence. All but one have an elevated post-void residual.

John (A)

John (A) has normal bladder capacity and mild increased bladder sensation. He has detrusor overactivity and urgency incontinence. His flow is reduced, but he generates a reasonably normal detrusor contraction and empties efficiently. His initial elevated PVR was a false positive.

John (B)

John (B) has markedly reduced bladder capacity and high pressure detrusor overactivity. He is urodynamically obstructed and has an elevated residual. His detrusor overactivity and de novo incontinence are likely neurogenic in origin, but chronic bladder outlet obstruction is another possibility.

John (C)

John (C) has a large capacity bladder with decreased bladder sensation. He has detrusor overactivity and leaks without awareness. He has a poorly contractile bladder causing an elevated residual. His

DHIC bladder may be a result of long-term bladder outlet obstruction or secondary to neurogenic bladder.

John (D)

John (D) has significant loss of bladder compliance associated with detrusor overactivity. He is urodynamically obstructed and has an elevated residual. His poor compliance is due to long-term obstruction and not from his stroke.

Diagnosis to treatment pathway

John (A-D) have a neurogenic bladder with de novo urinary incontinence. They have baseline BPH symptoms further complicating their presentation. Urodynamics are important in recommending their individual diagnosis to treatment pathway. Renal ultrasound and long-term surveillance is recommended in those with elevated residuals. Cystoscopy may assist when planning prostate surgery, and is used to diagnose a urethral stricture or an intravesical cause of the urinary incontinence.

We would like to make a few general statements regarding the management of patients like John (A–D) who are complicated and don't necessarily have a clear treatment path. In many cases, achieving symptom control is considered success, even if the PVR remains unchanged. If the patient can live with his chronic flow symptoms, then prostate surgery with its associated risks can likely be avoided. Medical therapy and cautiously advancing to more invasive OAB and BPH treatments is a good strategy.

- John (A–D) will be treated with alpha-adrenergic antagonists, hoping to improve symptoms and their PVR. Even partial benefit may justify their long-term use.

  With or without alpha-blockers, we would then recommend a β3-agonist or an antimuscarinic for persistent OAB. The risk of retention is higher in neurogenic men, especially those who are obstructed with an elevated residual. Having said that, the risk is surprisingly low, but long-term follow-up is important.

In those who fail medical therapy, the decision to follow the OAB versus the BPH diagnosis to treatment pathway is challenging and influenced by urodynamics. There are pros and cons to each approach, and having realistic treatment goals is important.

Sacral neuromodulation and PTNS are good options for refractory OAB in John (A–D). The risk of urinary retention with onabotulinumtoxinA in John (A) is similar to that of idiopathic men, since he is not obstructed and his stroke spared his voiding function. Even though John (A) has neurogenic detrusor overactivity, we would consider using the lower dose of 100 units. We would not recommend onabotulinumtoxinA to John (B–D), due to their increased risk of retention, unless they were willing to do CIC.

Recommending prostate surgery to John (A–D) is more controversial. Flow and residual is likely to improve in John (B) and (D), who are urodynamically obstructed from BPH. John (C)'s poorly contractile bladder is likely not going to respond favorably to a prostatectomy. John (A)'s flow may improve with surgery, but, in the absence of obstruction, his success rate is lower.

The primary risk of performing a prostatectomy is persistent or worsening OAB symptoms, especially in those with unfavorable bladder storage characteristics or neurogenic detrusor overactivity. Removing the proximal urethral sphincter may compromise continence. Patients with urgency and mild OAB symptoms can be converted to having urgency incontinence that sometimes is severe. Whether or not some of the minimally invasive prostate procedures are associated with a lower risk of incontinence is debatable.

Any symptom secondary to a stroke is usually not going to improve by relieving unrelated bladder outlet obstruction. Neurogenic storage symptoms may secondarily benefit from improved emptying but expectations must be guarded. This is especially the case with John (B), who has high pressure detrusor overactivity due to his stroke. Similarly, John (D)'s OAB symptoms are due to loss of bladder compliance, and will likely persist following prostatectomy.

Patients managed by prostatectomy and who experience persistent bothersome OAB can be successfully managed with refractory third-line therapies. Even onabotulinumtoxinA can be used in the now non-obstructed patient. The success of staged therapy is not guaranteed, and we caution against this treatment strategy.

CASE 2

Urinary Incontinence in Female with Multiple Sclerosis

Diagnosis

History

Jen is a 48-year-old female with multiple sclerosis who has urgency incontinence. She has very little warning and soaks 3 pads daily. She has foot-on-the-floor syndrome and gets up twice during the night to void. She has hourly frequency.

Her flow is slow and often associated with urgency. She has urinary hesitancy, her flow stops and starts, and she does not feel empty after urination.

Jen's multiple sclerosis has been stable for years. She has mild leg weakness but ambulates well. Her incontinence is impacting her work as a teacher.

Jen has a neurogenic bladder with urinary frequency, nocturia, and urgency incontinence. She has flow symptoms and was evaluated with urodynamics.

Physical exam

On pelvic examination the patient has mild urethral and bladder neck hypermobility and no SUI. She has no prolapse and her tissues were well estrogenized.

Post-void residual

88 mL

Urinalysis

Normal

Urodynamics

Jen (A)

During urodynamics, the patient had a MCC of 246 mL with increased bladder sensation. She had detrusor overactivity reaching pressures of 9 cmH$_2$O associated with mild urgency incontinence. She had no urodynamic SUI. During pressure flow, her P$_{det}$max was 28 cmH$_2$O and the Qmax was 16 mL/sec. The flow pattern was reasonably normal, and the EMG remained stable during voiding. The PVR was 86 mL (Figure M9-4).

M9-4: Jen (A) urodynamics

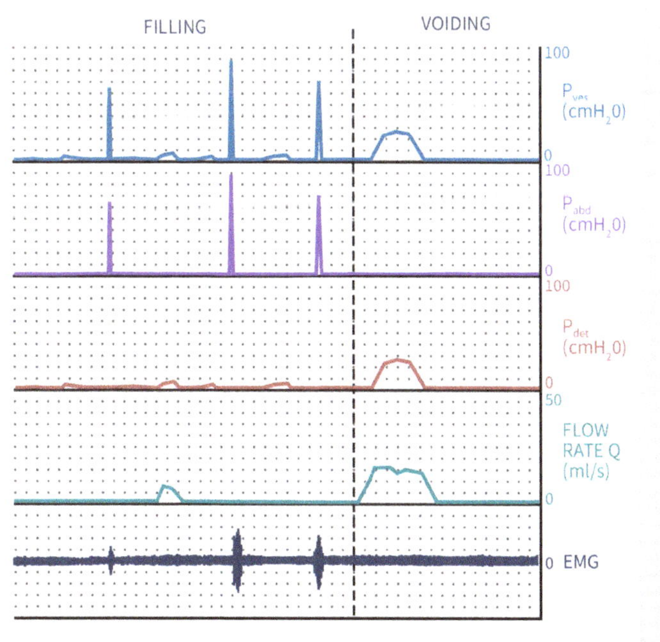

Jen (B)

During urodynamics, the patient had a MCC of 246 mL with increased bladder sensation. She had detrusor overactivity reaching pressures of 20 cmH_2O associated with urgency incontinence. She had no urodynamic SUI. She had difficulty initiating urination. She generated repetitive detrusor contractions of 7 cmH_2O associated with no flow. She finally voided with a P_{det}max of 38 cmH_2O and a Qmax of 6 mL/sec. The flow pattern was prolonged and intermittent. The increased EMG activity waxed and waned during voiding and the PVR was 87 mL (Figure M9-5).

Figure M9-5: Jen (B) urodynamics

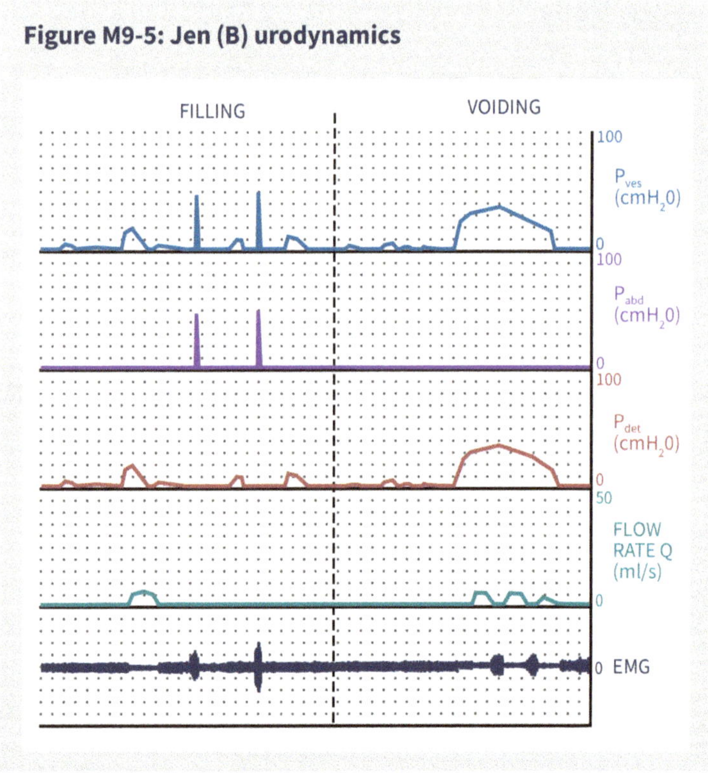

Jen (C)

During urodynamics, the patient had a MCC of 246 mL with increased bladder sensation. She had repetitive detrusor overactivity reaching pressures of 38 cmH$_2$O associated with urgency incontinence. She had no urodynamic SUI. During voiding, it was difficult to determine if she could void voluntarily. After several attempts, it was concluded that she was voiding off involuntary detrusor contractions reaching a pressure of 22 cmH$_2$O and a Qmax of 11 mL/sec. The flow pattern was mildly depressed, and the EMG increased during voiding. The PVR was 91 mL (Figure M9-6).

Figure M9-6: Jen (C) urodynamics

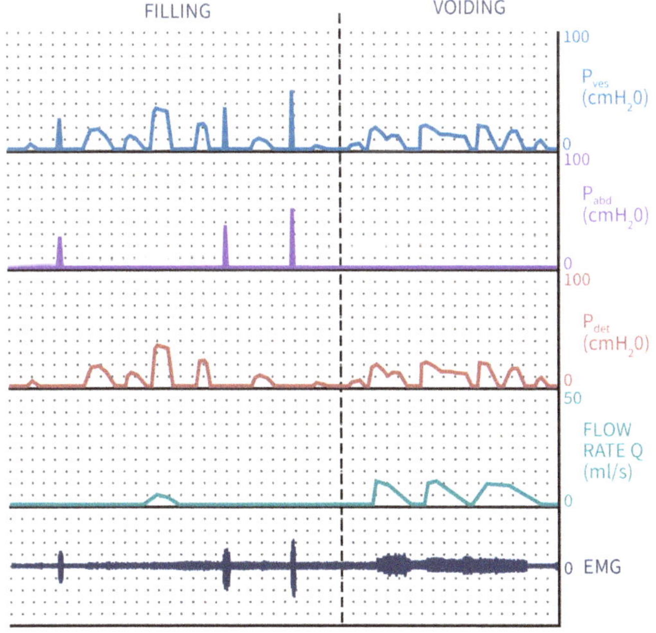

Jen (D)

During urodynamics, the patient had a MCC of 946 mL with decreased bladder sensation. She had low pressure detrusor overactivity reaching pressures of 8 cmH$_2$O associated with urgency incontinence. She had no urodynamic SUI. She could not generate a voluntary detrusor contraction, and voided by abdominal straining. The Qmax was 8 mL/sec and the EMG activity increased with straining. The PVR was 98 mL (Figure M9-7).

Figure M9-7: Jen (D) urodynamics

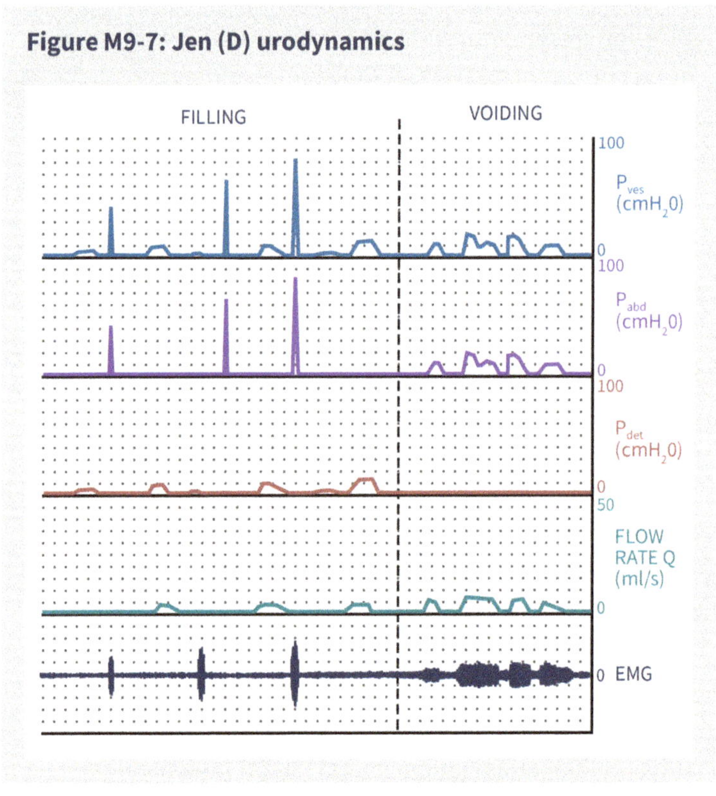

Diagnosis

Jen (A–D) have a neurogenic bladder secondary to multiple sclerosis. They have OAB symptoms with moderately severe urgency incontinence. They have flow symptoms with a PVR that is mildly elevated.

Jen (A)

Jen (A) has reduced bladder capacity and increased bladder sensation. She has low pressure detrusor overactivity associated with mild incontinence. Her pressure flow is reasonably normal, and her EMG activity was stable. Whether or not she would have mild detrusor sphincter dyssynergia if the EMG was measured by concentric needle electromyography is debatable.

Jen (B)

Jen (B) has a small capacity overactive detrusor associated with urgency incontinence. She has bladder outlet obstruction secondary to detrusor sphincter dyssynergia. Her urinary hesitancy with stopping and starting is secondary to intermittent DSD that commonly occurs in MS patients.

Jen (C)

Jen (C) has high pressure detrusor overactivity and unfavorable bladder storage characteristics. She is unable to void voluntarily and urinates off the top of an involuntary terminal contraction. On further questioning, Jen (C) reports that she normally voids when she experiences urgency. She does not think that she could otherwise urinate.

Jen (D)

Jen (D) has low pressure detrusor overactivity and urgency incontinence. She has a large capacity poorly contractile bladder which occurs in approximately 10% of symptomatic MS patients. Loosely speaking, she has DHIC secondary to a neurogenic bladder.

Diagnosis to treatment pathway

Approximately 78% of MS patients develop lower urinary tract symptoms ranging from overactive bladder to voiding symptoms and urinary retention. They most commonly have neurogenic detrusor overactivity with varying degrees of detrusor sphincter dyssynergia. A small percentage have a poorly contractile bladder, as the MS affects the pia mater of the sacral nerve simulating a peripheral lesion.

Urodynamics help define the bladder dysfunction and guide the diagnosis to treatment pathway. The evaluation also helps identify those at risk for developing renal deterioration secondary to high detrusor pressure.

Jen (A–D) have urgency incontinence and urinary flow symptoms. Their mildly elevated residual may be an early sign of this population's propensity towards incomplete bladder emptying and should be considered.

- We will manage Jen (A–D) primarily using the OAB diagnosis to treatment pathway. β3-agonists and antimuscarinics as monotherapy or in combination are effective in MS patients. Retention rates appear to be slightly higher with OAB medications, but which Jen is at greatest risk is unknown.
- An alpha-adrenergic antagonist is also reasonable to consider in an attempt to improve flow and post-void residual. Physical therapy may be effective in treating the lower urinary tract symptoms.

The urodynamic findings influence the recommendation of third-line therapies. We would offer Jen (A–D) sacral neuromodulation and PTNS to address the majority of their symptoms. Many patients symptomatically improve even if the PVR remains unchanged.

OnabotulinumtoxinA is FDA-approved for neurogenic detrusor overactivity and urgency incontinence in MS patients. Although its retention rate approaches 31%, the risk may vary according to the underlying bladder dysfunction. Jen (A) has reasonably normal voiding and her retention rate may be less. Jen (B)'s detrusor sphincter dyssynergia and Jen (D)'s poorly contractile bladder likely place them at higher risk. If Jen (C) truly voids off terminal involuntary detrusor contractions then she is at very high risk of developing retention with onabotulinumtoxinA. By eliminating her terminal DO, she would not be able to void. It is reasonable to consider using 100 units in patients at higher risk.

Jen (A–D) have a neurogenic bladder with a mildly elevated PVR. It's recommended to perform a renal ultrasound to assess renal health and to follow them long-term. This is especially important in Jen (C) who has a high pressure detrusor.

CASE 3

Urinary Incontinence in Male with Spinal Cord Injury

Diagnosis

History

Jack is a 47-year-old T8 paraplegic male with urinary incontinence dating back to an MVA 8 years earlier. He performs CIC four times daily and leaks in between catheterization. He wears two light pads during the day and has high volume enuresis.

Jack gets five UTI's per year that respond favorably to antibiotics. He has no past history of genitourinary surgery or renal calculi. He is on extended-release oxybutynin.

Prior to his accident Jack had normal bladder function.

Jack has a neurogenic bladder secondary to spinal cord injury. He has mild incontinence during the day and flooding bedwetting. He has recurrent UTI's and is on oxybutynin. He performs clean intermittent catheterization. He was evaluated with urodynamics and renal ultrasound.

Physical exam

On physical examination, his genitalia is normal. He has a 30-gram benign prostate. His neurologic exam is consistent with his complete neurologic injury. He has mild ankle edema.

Urinalysis

Few WBC's; rare bacteria (urine culture normal)

Renal ultrasound

Normal

Urodynamics

Jack (A)

During urodynamics, the patient had a MCC of 846 mL with no bladder sensation. He had detrusor overactivity reaching pressures of 9 cmH$_2$O and leaked a small amount not associated with awareness. Bladder compliance was normal. He had no urodynamic SUI and could not void voluntarily. EMG activity increased mildly during detrusor overactivity. Fluoroscopically, he had mild bladder trabeculation.

Jack (B)

During urodynamics, the patient had a MCC of 546 mL with no bladder sensation. He had detrusor overactivity reaching pressures of 69 cmH$_2$O and leaked a large amount not associated with awareness. His detrusor leak point pressure was 65 cmH$_2$O. Bladder compliance was normal, and he had no urodynamic SUI. He could not void voluntarily, and his EMG activity increased during detrusor overactivity. Fluoroscopically, he had a mild Christmas tree-shaped bladder, grade two left sided vesicoureteral reflux, and detrusor sphincter dyssynergia.

Jack (C)

During urodynamics, the patient had a MCC of 246 mL with no bladder sensation. He had detrusor overactivity reaching pressures of 12 cmH$_2$O and did not leak. Bladder compliance was decreased with an end filling pressure of 42 cmH$_2$O. At capacity, he leaked a large amount with a detrusor leak point pressure was 42 cmH$_2$O. He had no urodynamic SUI, and he could not void voluntarily. EMG activity remained stable during bladder filling. Fluoroscopically, he had a heavily trabeculated bladder and several small diverticula.

Diagnosis

Jack (A–C) have a neurogenic bladder with incomplete bladder emptying being managed by CIC. In spite of taking oxybutynin, they have urinary incontinence, especially at night. They have a history of recurrent UTI's.

Jack (A)

Jack (A) has a large capacity bladder and low pressure detrusor overactivity. He has mild external sphincter dyssynergia and a low detrusor leak point pressure. Fluoroscopically, his bladder looked reasonably normal.

Jack (B)

Jack (B) has normal bladder capacity and compliance. He has high pressure detrusor overactivity and a detrusor leak point pressure of 65 cmH$_2$O. He has external sphincter dyssynergia and fluoroscopic changes in keeping with a high pressure neurogenic bladder.

Jack (C)

Jack (C) has significantly reduced bladder capacity and low pressure detrusor overactivity. He has markedly reduced bladder compliance with a detrusor leak point pressure of 42 cmH$_2$O. The fluoroscopic findings are secondary to his neurogenic bladder.

Diagnosis to treatment pathway

Jack (A–C) have a neurogenic bladder and incomplete bladder emptying being managed with CIC. They have urinary incontinence that is especially severe at night. They have recurrent UTI's and are taking oxybutynin. The urodynamic findings are important in recommending their diagnosis to treatment pathway.

- Initially daily antibiotic prophylaxis may reduce UTI's, as well as downregulate symptoms and improve continence.
- Behavioral therapy is recommended in managing Jack (A–C). Reducing fluid intake later in the afternoon and catheterizing at bedtime can reduce enuresis. Dependent leg edema is common in spinal cord patients, and leg elevation during the day may lessen a nocturnal diuresis and improve continence. Catheter volumes should generally range between 300 and 700 mL. Consistent higher volumes may cause incontinence or elevated detrusor pressure.
- Catheterizing more frequently, combined with reasonable fluid intake, is an effective treatment to reduce urinary incontinence and high detrusor pressure. These strategies are especially important in Jack (B) and (C) who have high pressure bladders and elevated detrusor LPP's. Jack (A) has a low pressure bladder and can safely catheterize at high volumes.

Antimuscarinics and β-3 agonists are effective in managing urinary incontinence and reducing detrusor pressure. Switching to find the most effective agent, dose-escalation, and combining medications are excellent strategies.

OnabotulinumtoxinA is FDA-approved for urinary incontinence in spinal cord patients refractory to medical and behavioral therapy. Functional bladder capacity and detrusor pressure improve with 200 units. Higher dosages may be helpful in select cases.

Bladder augmentation increases functional capacity and reduces detrusor pressure. Antimuscarinics may still be required postoperatively to maximize efficacy. Patient compliance in performing CIC is a prerequisite, and long-term follow up is necessary.

Sacral neuromodulation and PTNS have no role in the management of complete spinal cord injured patients. Their effectiveness in those with partial lesions has been demonstrated.

Case 3 / Urinary incontinence in male with spinal cord injury

Long-term detrusor pressure monitoring and renal surveillance are important in spinal cord patients. Vesicourethral function can change over time, threatening bladder and renal health. Jack (A) has a large capacity low pressure system and is at lower risk. Jack (B) and (C) have high pressure detrusors that need more aggressive management and surveillance.

Nocturia and Nocturnal Enuresis: Diagnosis to Treatment Pathway

Nocturia is a highly prevalent and bothersome lower urinary tract symptom. The ICS defines it as the complaint that the individual has to wake at night one or more times to void. It has been established that getting up two or more times significantly impacts sleep and quality of life.

The majority of adults with nocturia have an underlying nocturnal polyuria (NP). NP is defined as a nocturnal urine output >33% of the daily total in patients older than 65 years and >20% in younger patients. Many of them have low levels of antidiuretic hormone, and their kidneys produce more urine at night. Others with congestive heart failure, dependent edema, uncontrolled diabetes, sleep apnea, and high fluid intake commonly have high nocturnal urine production.

Bladder diaries are important in diagnosing nocturia and other contributing factors. Many patients with NP also have a reduced functional bladder capacity. Diaries identify high fluid intake and the presence of global polyuria defined as a 24-hour urine volume of greater than 40 mL/kg.

Another common nighttime complaint is enuresis. With few exceptions, adult enuresis is secondary to an overactive detrusor and decreased sensory awareness that does not provoke awakening or immediate urinary loss upon awakening. Some of these patients are sedated from other medications. Having high-volume enuresis with only mild daytime symptoms is usually explained by an associated nocturnal diuresis. Other OAB patients wake up suddenly with urgency and experience foot-on-the-floor syndrome rushing to void. They may have less UUI during the day by responding sooner to their bladder signals.

Urodynamics play a role in the assessment of nighttime symptoms in select circumstances. Most patients have a 24-hour symptom complex that needs evaluation. Others have isolated symptoms, but their presentation is out of the ordinary or severe. In this diagnosis to treatment module, we will discuss the role of urodynamics in this population.

CASE 1

Elderly Woman with Nocturnal Enuresis

Diagnosis

History

Melissa is a 84-year-old woman with high volume bedwetting. She also experiences foot-on-floor syndrome and soaks two heavy Depends. She wears one pad during the day for mild mixed stress and urgency incontinence. She voids every one to two hours and gets up three times during the night to void.

Her flow is good, and she feels empty after urination.

She does not report urinary tract infections and has no neurologic risk factors. She uses a walker and has minimal medical comorbidities. She has not been treated for her voiding dysfunction.

Melissa is an elderly women with significant enuresis. She has a 24-hour symptom complex with mild mixed incontinence and overactive bladder. She has a functional component associated with her incontinence and was evaluated with urodynamics and cystoscopy.

Physical exam

On pelvic examination the patient has mild hypermobility of the bladder neck and no stress incontinence. She has moderate vaginal atrophy and narrowing of the introitus. She has no prolapse or peripheral edema.

Post-void residual urine volume

12 mL

Urinalysis

Few WBC's, rare bacteria.

Cystoscopy

Normal. No evidence of occult cystitis.

Urodynamics

Melissa (A)

During urodynamics, the patient had a MCC of 482 mL with normal bladder sensation. During filling, she had detrusor overactivity reaching a pressure of 21 cmH_2O associated with moderate urgency incontinence. She had no urodynamic SUI generating pressures of 130 cmH_2O. Her pressure flow and EMG were normal (Figure M10-1).

Figure M10-1: Melissa (A) urodynamics

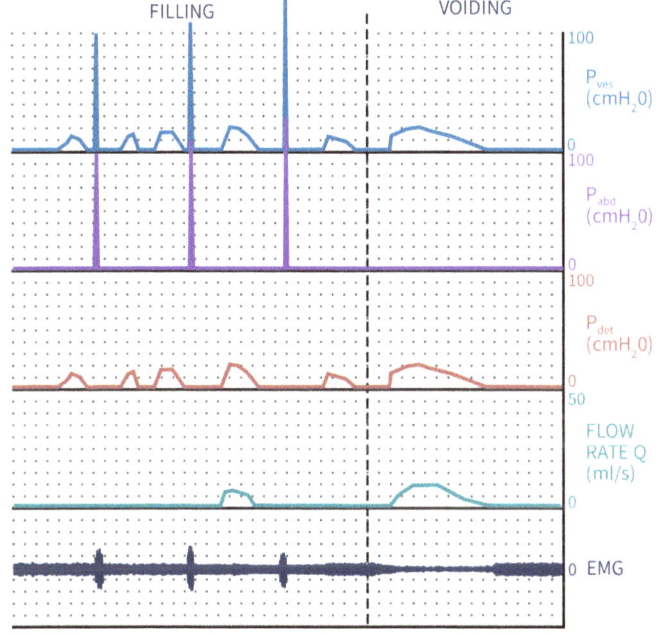

Melissa (B)

During urodynamics, the patient had a MCC of 482 mL with normal bladder sensation. During filling, she had detrusor overactivity reaching a pressure of 6 cmH$_2$O and no incontinence. She had significant urodynamic SUI with a leak point pressure of 12 cmH$_2$O. Her pressure flow and EMG were normal (Figure M10-2).

Figure M10-2: Melissa (B) urodynamics

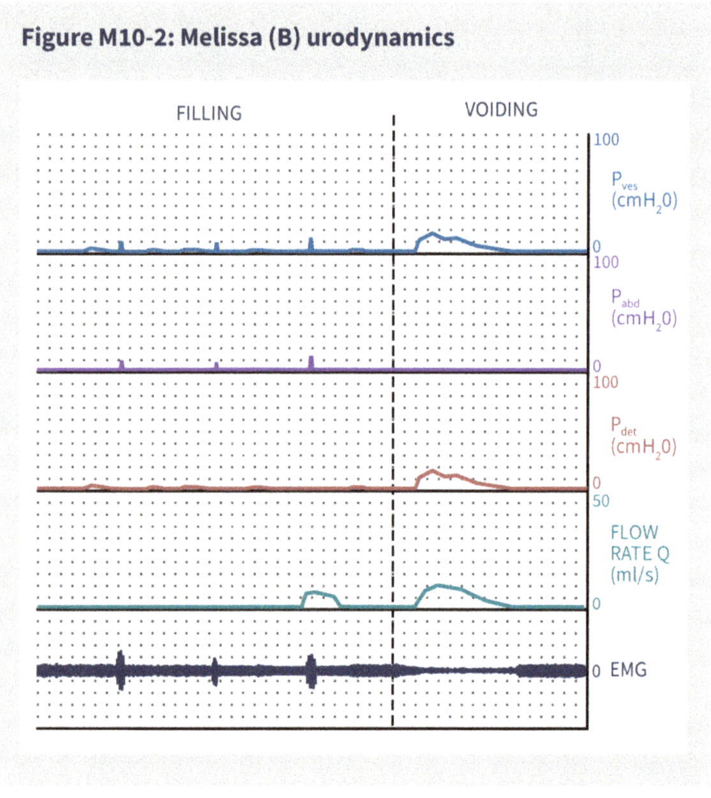

Diagnosis

Melissa (A) and (B) have high volume enuresis and mild mixed incontinence. They have OAB with nighttime frequency and use a walker to ambulate.

Melissa (A)

Melissa (A) has detrusor overactivity associated with moderately severe urgency incontinence. She has no urodynamic SUI even at higher abdominal pressures.

Melissa (B)

Melissa (B) has low pressure detrusor overactivity and significant urodynamic SUI with intrinsic sphincter deficiency.

Diagnosis to treatment pathway

Melissa (A) and (B) primarily have nocturnal enuresis and nocturia. They have milder daytime symptoms with mixed incontinence. Their diagnosis to treatment pathway is influenced by their urodynamic evaluation.

Melissa (A)

- Melissa (A) will be treated using the OAB diagnosis to treatment pathway. Her 24-hour symptom complex is primarily from detrusor overactivity, and her SUI is mild.

  We will manage her with behavioral therapy and OAB medication. Bladder retraining during the day can positively influence nighttime symptoms. Women who wake up with urgency are instructed to perform a "quick flick" Kegel before rising out of bed in an attempt to abort overactivity and reduce foot-on-the-floor syndrome. Fluid modifications can also be beneficial.
- If Melissa (A) fails medication, she will be offered third-line OAB therapies. Based on her age and functional status, PTNS will likely be her recommended treatment. OnabotulinumtoxinA and SNM are effective but may be less ideal in her case.

- Desmopressin could play a distant role in treating Melissa (A). The literature supports that approximately 80% of adults who get up two or more times at night to urinate have a nocturnal diuresis. It may be difficult to measure her nighttime urine output because of her enuresis. Desmopressin is associated with hyponatremia especially in the elderly.

Melissa (B)

- Melissa (B) will be treated similarly, knowing that she also has ISD. She will be managed symptomatically, but OAB therapies may be less effective because of her urethral dysfunction. She might have reported more severe stress incontinence if she was active.
- If she fails medical and behavioral therapy, Melissa (B) has two reasonable choices. We would offer PTNS, but, based on her ISD, a urethral bulking agent could be effective. Successful treatment with either one sometimes converts enuresis to experiencing increased nocturia and foot-on-the-floor syndrome. These partial responders may improve by reintroducing OAB agents that were previously mildly successful. Combining OAB agents with neuro-modulation is an effective strategy in treating enuresis.

Many patients like Melissa have other medical conditions including uncontrolled diabetes mellitus, congestive heart failure, sleep apnea, and peripheral edema. Managing these can significantly impact nighttime symptoms.

Young Woman with Nocturnal Enuresis

Diagnosis

History

Tara is a 21-year-old woman with primary enuresis. She wets the bed nightly dating back to childhood. As a young teen, she failed an alarm mat and medication. She is a deep sleeper and has no family history of enuresis.

She voids every 3 hours during the day and has no nocturia. Her flow is intermittent, and she feels empty after urination. Sometimes she has urgency but no urgency incontinence.

She has no neurologic risk factors or symptoms and has infrequent urinary tract infections. She is sexually active and is self-conscious about her incontinence.

Tara is a young woman with enuresis. She has minimal daytime voiding dysfunction with mild flow symptoms and intermittent urgency. Primary enuresis is highly prevalent in children with approximately 6% wetting the bed at age 6. About 15% outgrow the condition annually with 1% still having the problem in adulthood. We view persistent enuresis in adults as a presentation out of the ordinary and routinely order urodynamics in this population.

Physical exam

On pelvic examination, the patient has a well-supported bladder neck and no stress incontinence. She has normal perineal sensation, no stigmata of spina bifida occulta, and a palpable sacrum.

Post-void residual urine volume

2 mL

Urinalysis

Normal

Urodynamics

Tara (A)

During urodynamics, the patient had a MCC of 412 mL with mild increased bladder sensation. During filling, she had detrusor overactivity reaching a pressure of 11 cmH_2O associated with urgency but no urgency incontinence. She had no urodynamic SUI generating pressures of 160 cmH_2O. Her pressure flow and EMG were normal (Figure M10-3).

Figure M10-3: Tara (A) urodynamics

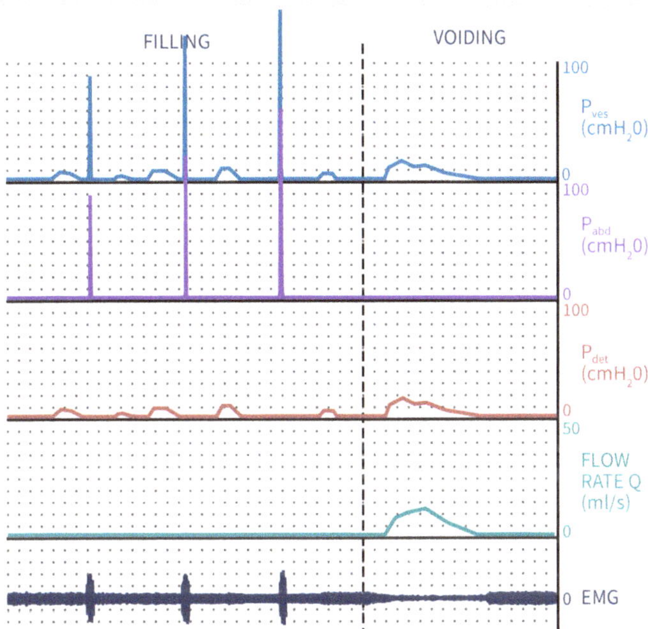

Tara (B)

During urodynamics, the patient had a MCC of 512 mL with normal bladder sensation. During filling, she had no detrusor overactivity or urodynamic SUI. Her pressure flow and EMG were normal (Figure M10-4).

Figure M10-4: Tara (B) urodynamics

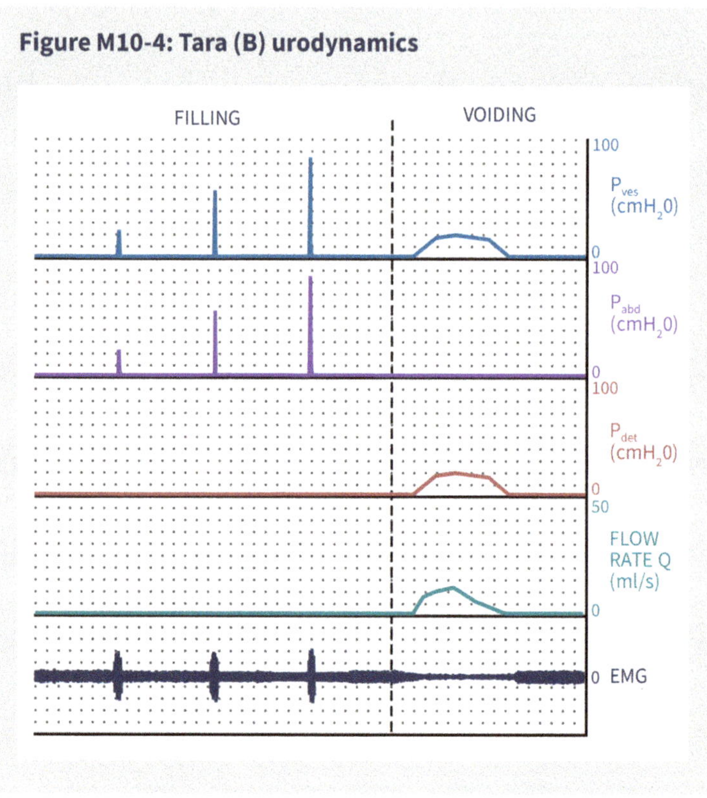

Tara (C)

During urodynamics, the patient had a MCC of 189 mL and increased bladder sensation. She had loss of bladder compliance with an end filling pressure of 28 cmH$_2$O. She had low pressure detrusor overactivity associated with urgency. She had urodynamic SUI leaking a few drops at 106 cmH$_2$O. During voiding, she voided 180 mL with a P$_{det}$max of 30 cmH$_2$O and the Qmax was 6 mL/sec. Her flow pattern was prolonged and intermittent. The EMG variably increased during voiding. During fluoroscopy, her bladder was heavily trabeculated with a small left-sided diverticulum. She had bilateral grade two vesicoureteral reflux. During voiding, she had obstruction at the level of the rhabdosphincter.

Tara (D)

During urodynamics, the patient had a MCC of 300 mL associated with increased bladder sensation. She had impressive detrusor overactivity reaching pressures of 44 cmH$_2$O. It took several moments for her to abort the contractions and she did not leak. She had no urodynamic SUI. During voiding, she voided 180 mL with a P$_{det}$max of 41 cmH$_2$O and the Qmax was 12 mL/sec. EMG activity increased during voiding. Fluoroscopically, she had a normal appearing smooth bladder. During voiding, she had obstruction at the level of the rhabdosphincter or pelvic floor.

Diagnosis

Tara (A–D) have primary enuresis. They have mild daytime flow symptoms and sometimes experience urgency.

Tara (A)

Tara (A) has a mildly reduced bladder capacity and increased bladder sensation. She has an overactive detrusor and no SUI. She has normal voiding.

Tara (B)

Tara (B) has normal bladder filling and emptying. She has no detrusor overactivity or urodynamic SUI. Her study is within normal limits.

Tara (C)

Tara (C) has markedly reduced bladder capacity and loss of compliance. She has low pressure detrusor overactivity and mild urodynamic SUI. She had external sphincter dyssynergia and is obstructed at the level of the rhabdosphincter.

Tara (D)

Tara (D) has significantly reduced bladder capacity and increased bladder sensation. She has high pressure detrusor overactivity and no incontinence. She has high pressure voiding and her obstruction is at the level of the rhabdosphincter or pelvic floor.

Diagnosis to treatment pathway

Tara (A–D) have nocturnal enuresis and mild daytime symptoms. Based on urodynamics, there are differences in their individual diagnosis to treatment pathway.

Tara (A)

Tara (A)'s enuresis is due to detrusor overactivity. She has favorable bladder storage characteristics and no evidence of neurogenic bladder dysfunction or obstruction.

- She will be managed with the OAB diagnosis to treatment pathway. Behavioral therapy with fluid modifications will be emphasized. Antimuscarinics and β3 agonists will be recommended and used in combination when clinically indicated.
- Imipramine and desmopressin that are commonly prescribed for pediatric enuresis are other options. Young adults have less nocturnal polyuria but may still respond to desmopressin.

- If Tara (A) fails medical therapy she will be offered third-line OAB therapies. We are biased toward sacral neuromodulation, although onabotulinumtoxinA and PTNS are effective options. All three refractory therapies are less ideal in younger patients.

Tara (B)

Tara (B) has the same diagnosis and underlying pathophysiology. In spite of her having normal urodynamics, her enuresis is due to detrusor overactivity even though it was not demonstrated. She has no other vesicourethral dysfunction to explain her symptoms. Her diagnosis to treatment pathway will be identical to Tara (A).

Tara (C)

Tara (C) has enuresis, and her video-urodynamics highly suggest the diagnosis of neurogenic bladder. She has unfavorable bladder storage characteristics with detrusor overactivity and loss of bladder compliance. She is obstructed at the level of the rhabdosphincter, which is pathognomonic. She has occult mild urodynamic SUI, which may be secondary to urethral sphincter denervation.

In the absence of finding an underlying neurologic etiology, some might diagnose Tara (C) as having Hinman syndrome or non-neurogenic neurogenic bladder. These patients are functionally obstructed by habitually contracting their pelvic floor during voiding. Hinman syndrome or non-neurogenic neurogenic bladder is another term for dysfunctional voiding, but has been regarded as obsolete by the International Children Continence Society.

- First and foremost, Tara (C) will be referred for a thorough neurologic evaluation. A baseline renal ultrasound will be obtained to rule out the presence of hydronephrosis. She will be followed with annual imaging, and her urodynamics will be repeated intermittently to reassess bladder pressure.

- Tara (C) will be managed similar to the first two patients. Patients with neurogenic bladder may experience poor flow with OAB medication, but retention is rare. Although unproven, behavioral therapy may be less effective in those with neurogenic bladder.
- She will be offered third-line OAB therapies if conservative treatments fail. Based on the literature, her risk of retention requiring CIC approaches 30% with onabotulinumtoxinA if she does have a neurogenic bladder. Sacral neuromodulation and PTNS eliminate this risk.

Tara (D)

Tara (D) has high pressure detrusor overactivity, decreased bladder capacity, and high pressure voiding. Her bladder storage characteristics are somewhat unfavorable and out of the ordinary for a young patient with idiopathic OAB. Whether or not to refer her to neurology is based on index of suspicion. In the absence of having more worrisome urodynamic finding, the majority of neurologic evaluations in these circumstances are normal. A renal ultrasound is reasonable to consider as another safety measure.

- Without a neurologic diagnosis, Tara (D)'s detrusor overactivity and high pressure obstructed voiding are likely due to pelvic floor dyssynergia. She will be managed similar to Tara (A) and (B), and pelvic floor therapy will be emphasized. If medical and behavioral therapy fail, then third-line treatments will be recommended. Unproven, the risk of retention with onabotulinumtoxinA may be greater based on her pelvic floor dyssynergia, and sacral neuromodulation is an excellent choice.

Underactive Bladder: Diagnosis to Treatment Pathway

The underactive bladder (UAB) is defined by the ICS as a detrusor contraction of reduced strength and/or duration, resulting in prolonged bladder emptying and/or failure to achieve complete bladder emptying within a normal time span. It's a urodynamic diagnosis typically associated with diminished bladder sensation and elevated residual.

The causes of UAB are often classified as myogenic, neuropathic, pharmacologic, and aging. Many men with chronic bladder outlet obstruction and patients with diabetes have myogenic failure. Bladder acontractility is common in patients with neurogenic bladder dysfunction. A number of medications and aging can adversely affect detrusor function.

Patients with UAB usually report obstructive symptoms or have overactive bladder symptoms due to incomplete bladder emptying. Secondary effects include urinary tract infections, vesicoureteral reflux, and hydronephrosis.

In this module, we will limit our discussion to idiopathic underactive bladder in women. Poor detrusor function in other patient types will be discussed elsewhere.

CASE 1

Young Woman with Urinary Retention

Diagnosis

History

Jill is a 26-year-old woman who presents with urinary retention. She has a 10 month history of poor flow, hesitancy, and straining to urinate. Her flow stops and starts, and she does not feel empty after urination. Recently, she starting voiding every 45 minutes and getting up twice during the night to urinate. Sometimes she stands in the shower in order to initiate urination.

She is continent and has no neurologic risk factors or symptoms. She has not had previous bladder or pelvic surgery and has no history of UTI's.

Jill has no other complicating urologic factors, is medically healthy, and has not been treated for her voiding dysfunction.

Jill has significant flow symptoms associated with an overactive bladder. Her presentation is out of the ordinary, and she was evaluated with urodynamics and cystoscopy.

Physical exam

On pelvic examination, the patient has mild urethral and bladder neck hypermobility and no SUI. She has no evidence of vaginitis, urethral diverticulum, Skene's gland cyst, or meatal stenosis. She has normal vaginal and perineal sensation, no stigmata of spina bifida occulta, and a palpable sacrum.

Post-void residual urine volume

712 mL

Urinalysis

Normal

Cystoscopy

Normal

Urodynamics

During urodynamics, the patient had a MCC of 1100 mL associated with decreased bladder sensation. She has no involuntary detrusor overactivity or urodynamic SUI. During voiding, she generated a fleeting detrusor contraction with a P_{det}max of 6 cmH$_2$O and a Qmax of 4 mL/sec. She intermittently strained to urinate voiding small amounts. Her EMG activity increased with straining, and the PVR was 742 mL. During fluoroscopy the bladder contour was normal, and she had no vesicoureteral reflux (Figure M11-1).

Figure M11-1: Jill urodynamics

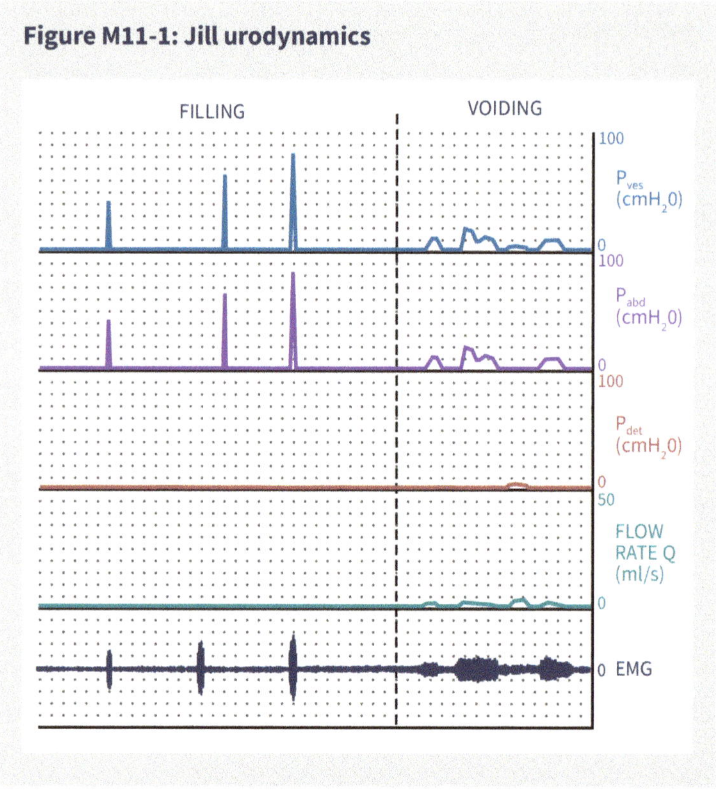

Diagnosis

Jill has impressive flow and OAB symptoms with a markedly elevated PVR. Based on her residual, she had a renal ultrasound that was normal.

She has a large capacity bladder associated with decreased bladder sensation. Her voiding pressure is low and poorly sustained, resulting in incomplete bladder emptying. She has no urodynamic evidence of bladder outlet obstruction or neurogenic bladder.

Diagnosis to treatment pathway

Jill has complicated voiding dysfunction and impressive urinary retention. Her recent increase in frequency is from incomplete bladder emptying and probably represents worsening of a chronic bladder disorder.

In the absence of other causes, Jill has idiopathic non-obstructed urinary retention. It's a poorly understood condition and challenging to treat.

Concentric needle EMG of the external sphincter divides these patients into two categories. Those who demonstrate complex repetitive discharge are referred to as having Fowler's Syndrome, while patients who show no activity have idiopathic urinary retention. This differentiation is difficult and probably has little clinical relevance.

Fowler's syndrome is commonly seen in women with polycystic ovary syndrome and endometriosis. Typically, in the third decade, they present with retention with residuals greater than one liter. They have no underlying neurologic or urologic disorder. It's believed that excessive excitability of the external urethral sphincter may prevent its adequate relaxation necessary for voiding.

Chronic urinary retention in healthy women is managed similar to DHIC patients. Symptomatic management, improving emptying, and minimizing complications are the goals of therapy. Spontaneous recovery sometimes occurs, especially in younger patients with precipitating factors such as post-pelvic surgery and postpartum.

Conservative strategies include scheduled voiding, gentle Valsalva or Credé maneuver, and pelvic floor physical therapy. Alpha-adrenergic antagonists can be helpful in a minority.

We don't offer the acetylcholine agonist bethanecol because of its lack of efficacy. We often recommend clean intermittent catheterization, which can be effective in reducing symptoms and minimizing UTI's associated with elevated residuals. Even catheterizing once or twice daily can make a positive impact.

Sacral neuromodulation is FDA-approved for non-obstructive urinary retention. It has been shown to be more effective in women than men and is also beneficial in those with Fowler's syndrome. We discourage SNM in older men who have myogenic failure secondary to chronic bladder outlet obstruction and aging.

New therapies for UAB are currently being investigated. Medications targeting prostaglandin E2 and EP2 receptors are under development. The authors have injected onabotulinumtoxinA into the urethral sphincter, which has shown promise in reducing lower urinary tract symptoms and PVR. Future treatments for UAB will likely include stem cell regenerative technology and gene therapy.

Behavioral therapy, alpha-adrenergic antagonists, sacral nerve stimulation, and CIC are the treatment options for idiopathic non-obstructive urinary retention. Symptomatic improvement is considered a success even if the PVR remains unchanged. Long-term surveillance for the development of silent hydronephrosis or escalating PVR's is recommended. Antibiotic prophylaxis is effective in managing recurrent UTI's.

Looking Forward: Ambulatory Urodynamic Monitoring (AUM)

For years, I've wanted to write *The Art of LUTS*, and I appreciate my friend David Staskin, MD for editing the book, while still allowing me to share my thoughts and experience. As the book comes to completion, it's fitting to once again thank David for his expertise and willingness to help me deliver the best product.

In our discussion regarding ambulatory urodynamics, David cleverly compared the utilization of cystometry and ambulatory urodynamic monitoring (AUM) in the evaluation of LUTS to a cardiologist measuring the electrical activity of the heart using an electrocardiogram (ECG) versus a Holter monitor. Although the ECG is the gold standard in diagnosing many cardiac diseases, false negatives occur, and further evaluation is necessary. The Holter evaluates electrical activity for 24 hours or longer, and detects arrhythmias that go undiagnosed during the shorter study.

One could argue that the provocative maneuvers used during CMG are the exercise stress test of conventional UDS, but they can still miss bladder dysfunctions only detected during AUM and while the patient is performing their normal activity. And as is the case in cardiology, diagnosing DO, SUI, or for example, a high detrusor leak point pressure during prolonged observation may be clinically relevant.

Ambulatory urodynamic monitoring

The International Continence Society defines ambulatory urodynamic monitoring as any functional test of the lower urinary tract predominantly using natural antegrade filling of the bladder and reproducing the patient's normal activity that is likely going to provoke their symptoms. It offers a longer and more physiological assessment of the bladder, urethra, and pelvic floor.

Many consider AUM to be valuable in investigating lower urinary tract dysfunction in patients with LUTS and who have inconclusive results on conventional urodynamics. Although ambulatory studies have been demonstrated to be more sensitive than cytometry, there remains no clear consensus about their role in clinical practice.

My experience with ambulatory urodynamics dates back to my fellowship in Sheffield, England with my dear friend, Professor Chris Chapple. I remember Dr. Derek Rosario and myself pulling the Medical Measurement System (MMS) unit out of the box for the first time and attaching it to our study patient. It was an intriguing and enlightening experience for all.

Ambulatory studies generally take 3–4 hours, or at least capture one bladder filling and voiding cycle. Air-filled or microtip catheters are inserted into the bladder and rectal canal, and securely taped adjacent to the anus and external urethral meatus to reduce dislodgement and to minimize movement artifacts. After dressing, the catheters are connected to the recording device, which can be carried using a shoulder strap.

Patients are instructed to drink plenty of fluids and to perform activities known to reproduce troublesome symptoms. An electronic pad, an event marker button, or a bladder diary are used to record urinary leakage. Ultrasound measures the post-void residual urine volume and the use of prophylactic antibiotics is optional.

AUM – what do we know?

For decades, dedicated clinician scientists have studied ambulatory urodynamics in asymptomatic patients and in men and women with lower urinary tract symptoms. Most commonly, the diagnostic capability of AUM has been assessed in those having had previous nondiagnostic traditional studies. It's well accepted that urodynamics often doesn't reproduce the patient's symptoms, or it identifies symptoms that are not present under normal circumstances.

In *The Art of LUTS*, I purposely kept literature citations to a minimum and will continue to do so. Although the ambulatory data is modest and increasing, there is little study consistency, the number of patients studied is small, and the best monitoring technique has not yet been agreed upon. Having said that, I think there are a number of things that the literature supports and that we can confidently say about ambulatory urodynamics.

AUM is more sensitive than cystometry in detecting detrusor overactivity and SUI in women with urinary incontinence.

Multiple studies demonstrate that AUM may diagnose detrusor overactivity (DO) and SUI in women with urinary incontinence that went undetected during conventional urodynamics. Reported rates of nondiagnostic cystometry vary from 19 to 44%, with a false-negative rate for detecting DO approaching 50% in some studies.

The reason for this is likely related to the duration of one study versus the other, and the presence of the guarding reflex, which is more common in apprehensive patients, and exacerbated by the unnatural lab setting. Voluntary or involuntary contraction of the pelvic floor and urethral sphincter may secondarily suppress bladder activity during bladder filling, and maintain continence during Valsalva. Although provocative maneuvers are used with cystometry to elicit DO and SUI, the real-world activities during AUM may be more effective. In addition, the rapid filling rate associated with urodynamics might temporarily subdue the expression of DO resulting in a negative test, while in others it may stimulate a false-positive.

Asymptomatic women demonstrate detrusor overactivity during ambulatory studies.

Asymptomatic women commonly demonstrate DO during ambulatory urodynamics, with an incidence in some studies ranging between 33–69%. The number and amplitude of the overactive contractions varied amongst individuals. It would be naïve to think that putting the key into the door, running water, high bladder volumes, or certain foods and beverages wouldn't trigger an involuntary detrusor contraction in normal individuals. Think of the number of times that you may have experienced urinary urgency during a normal day, but clinically you do not have an overactive bladder.

AUM is valuable in assessing voiding efficiency in men with LUTS.

A number of studies have demonstrated that the voiding detrusor pressure is higher during AUM versus conventional cystometry, but the proportion of men classified as being obstructed, equivocal, and non-obstructed does not appear to differ significantly.

One investigator demonstrated that a high percentage of men with voiding complaints, and who were diagnosed as having an acontractile bladder during cystometry, generated a voluntary detrusor contraction during ambulatory monitoring. Again, it has been postulated that the fast filling rate during cytometry may cause rapid stretching of the detrusor muscle and adversely affect contractility, or an increased guarding reflex, sometimes referred to as "bashful bladder," may be the explanation.

AUM is an effective tool used in the evaluation of patients with neurogenic bladder dysfunction, especially those at risk of developing hydronephrosis.

It's well recognized that the rapid filling rate of CMG may negatively impact detrusor compliance, especially in those with neurogenic bladder. Experts believe that the physiologic filling rate associated with AUM provides a more accurate measurement of bladder pressure, thereby reducing the risk of over diagnosing decreased bladder compliance. AUM has also been shown to be more sensitive in detecting neurogenic detrusor overactivity in this population.

As a result, AUM appears to be an excellent diagnostic tool to assess neurogenic patients, especially those at risk of developing hydrone-phrosis, with or without vesicoureteral reflux. AUM studies have demonstrated that a chronically elevated detrusor pressure between contractions, as well as frequent, high amplitude, long duration detrusor contractions during bladder storage, and a high post-void residual urine volume likely precipitates hydronephrosis.

AUM may alter the diagnosis to treatment pathway in LUTS patients by identifying underlying pathophysiology not detected by cystometry.

Multiple studies have investigated the usefulness of AUM in evaluating LUTS patients with nondiagnostic conventional urodynamics, and whose symptoms were not reproduced. Without elaborating, many investigators altered their diagnosis to treatment pathway as a result of the ambulatory findings.

For example, detecting detrusor overactivity or SUI not otherwise detected during CMG may alter the diagnosis to treatment pathway, especially in women with mixed urinary incontinence. Demonstrating detrusor contractility in men with urinary retention initially diagnosed as having an acontractile bladder could dramatically change treatment. And knowledge of the minute by minute detrusor pressure in a patient with neurogenic bladder dysfunction could have therapeutic impact, versus following them with conventional studies.

AUM - where are we going?

First generation AUM technology requires urethral and rectal catheters similar to office-based testing that are attached to a portable recording device. Study interpretation may be time consuming and relies upon patient reporting of events in order to best interpret the study.

Ambulatory systems are sometimes plagued by technical issues including device failure, data loss, and catheter displacement. Well-trained nurses insert and fix the catheters correctly and instruct patients thoroughly.

Novel AUM devices using wireless, catheter-free, battery-powered systems to monitor bladder pressure are currently being developed. The Glean Urodynamics System (GUS) is an intravesical AUM device that conducts standard urodynamic testing including uroflowmetry, cystometry, urethral pressure profile, and micturition studies, and is seeking FDA approval in 2025.

Glean is a long, flexible, disposable sensor that is inserted into the bladder via the urethra using an insertion tool, and then curls unanchored into a circular shape to avoid migrating into the bladder neck (Figure 17.1). The sensor monitors bladder pressure for extended periods of time, and is easily removed by pulling a removal string. The data is then downloaded and interpreted.

Figure 17. 1 Glean Urodynamics System

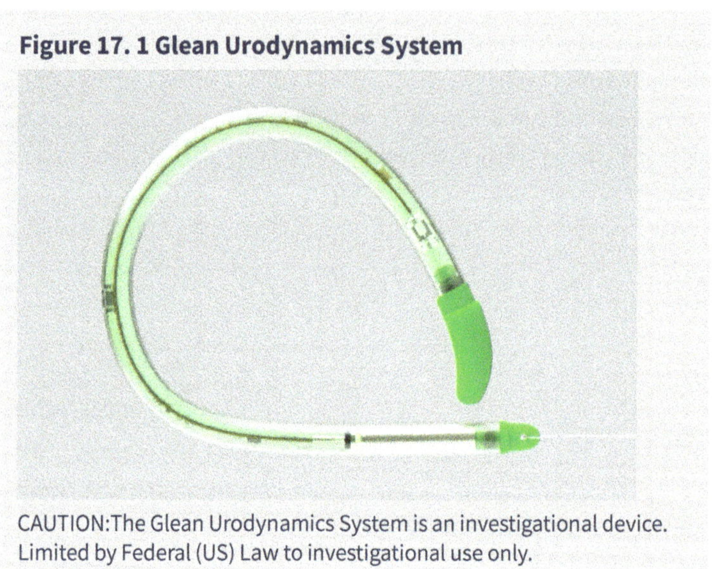

CAUTION:The Glean Urodynamics System is an investigational device. Limited by Federal (US) Law to investigational use only.

Catheter-free, single-channel, pressure monitoring devices like Glean assume that intravesical pressure alone is sufficient to characterize bladder function. Although early data suggests that this will provide reliable urodynamic information, limitations might include artifacts from patient movement or changes in abdominal pressure misinterpreted as increases in detrusor pressure. Others have developed mathematical algorithms to reduce abdominal pressure artefacts, hoping to produce data comparable to that of catheter-based urodynamics. In future generations of Glean, an abdominal pressure sensor and the ability to measure bladder volume in real time will be available.

Clinical perspective

When I moved to the US to begin my academic career, I purchased an ambulatory urodynamic system. I had no intention of using it clinically but only as a research tool. I felt that the functionality of AUM was inferior to my state-of-the-art video-urodynamics lab, and it was too cumbersome for clinical practice.

Recognizing that I have not clinically used Glean or similar technology, I would like to discuss how future ambulatory systems may benefit us in diagnosing and treating patients with lower urinary tract symptoms. My comments will assume that these new technologies will provide accurate uroflowmetry, cystometry, and pressure flow studies, and that patients are able to correctly record necessary events during the monitoring period. Ideally, the patients should be evaluated for up to 24 hours or longer, and be able to perform activities that elicit their symptoms. The downloaded data must be easily and rapidly interpreted, with acceptable sensitivity and specificity. And finally, AUM systems must be simple to implement, cost-effective, well tolerated, and safe.

As discussed in Chapter 3, I consider patient features, how well the bladder stores, how incompetent is the outlet, and voiding efficiency when evaluating LUTS patients. I use the history, physical, often urodynamics, and sometimes cystoscopy, to analyze each one of them. I'm excited that AUM may augment conventional studies, or replace them in many patients.

New technologies will minimize the need of having an expert UDS nurse or finding a "Brenda" to ensure accurate studies. By eliminating some of the well-known physician and patient barriers associated with cystometry, ambulatory devices may open the door to urodynamics to the thousands of clinicians currently not performing them.

If effective, I'm also hopeful that AUM will be used sooner in the diagnostic process, with physicians considering it as one of their diagnostic stethoscopes in many patients. Imagine following the history and physical examination, and measuring the uroflow and PVR, placing the Glean Urodynamic System, and asking the patient to return the following day to download the information. This would dramatically augment the physician's understanding of the patient's bladder dysfunction, and allow for early establishment of an effective diagnosis to treatment pathway.

Patient features

Patient features are important, as they may contribute to symptoms and influence diagnosis and treatment. Their clinical relevance is independent of the type of urodynamics utilized. When it comes to ambulatory monitoring, it's ideal that the patient has the functional and cognitive ability to record bladder events in order to maximize the accuracy and clinical benefit of the study. This is commonly performed using an app on a smart phone.

The patient generated marked events, which, when superimposed on the cystometric recording, help define the vesicouethral dysfunction in real time and allow the clinician to relive the patient's subjective experience. The event markers should be easy to use, hit the sweet spot in their complexity, and ideally the app should include an ecosystem providing patients the ability to communicate in greater detail.

The ecosystem could send regular messages or signals encouraging the patient to summarize what they have experienced in the last several hours. Retrospectively, they could add granularity to a marked event, make comments regarding events that went unmarked, and put into context what they were doing when the event occurred. It would be easy for patients to record the number and types of pads utilized and whether they were damp, moderately wet, or soaked.

For example, imagine a patient being able to dictate or text that in the last several hours they experienced two episodes of urgency incontinence, both triggered while getting out of a chair, and soaking their Depends. And that they also leaked a few drops with a sneeze, but it was the high volume episodes associated with urgency that were most bothersome. This would be much more valuable than only seeing two overactive detrusor contractions and an SUI event marked on the cystometrogram in the assessment of a woman with mixed incontinence.

An ecosystem that blended cystometry and its event markings with the patient's recall of their bladder experience, could revolutionize the diagnostic assessment of LUTS patients. And with the help of artificial intelligence, it would be valuable if the patient's input could be readily placed into the medical record as an easy to read descriptive notation.

Especially in the age of using rushed, less descriptive history templates, and knowing that the bladder is an unreliable witness, AUM, combined with a patient interactive ecosystem, would be a tremendous addition to the diagnostic armamentarium.

How well does the bladder store?

The most comprehensive assessment of bladder storage includes the history, the voiding diary, and filling cystometry, either measured with conventional or ambulatory studies. One of the advantages of AUM is that it automatically generates an electronic diary and has the potential of including an ecosystem augmenting the history.

Favorable and unfavorable cystometric patterns demonstrated during conventional CMG help define the severity of the bladder storage disorder, which can impact treatment recommendations and outcome. It will be interesting to see if ambulatory studies reproduce the findings or if they redefine the bladder's storage capability. Rapid filling during CMG can trigger overactivity, while in some it may temporarily suppress the expression of DO, giving a false negative.

Monitoring for extended periods of time, especially while performing stimulating activities, has the potential of best defining bladder storage and differentiating one patient from the other. For example, having a few low pressure overactive detrusor contractions detected over several hours and associated with urgency is different than the presence of multiple high-pressure contractions occurring several times per hour and associated with severe urgency incontinence.

Future ambulatory analysis will be able to provide a number of CMG measurements, including bladder sensation and capacity, the number and pressure of overactive detrusor contractions, the severity of incontinence associated with DO, and bladder compliance. Total study analysis in combination with predetermined segmented analyses would be beneficial. Concentrating on specific time frames may identify symptoms that are more severe or bothersome during certain periods and activities, as well as help evaluate nighttime events.

How incompetent is the outlet?

The assessment of bladder neck and urethral function is best determined by the history, physical, and urodynamics. Regardless of whether conventional or ambulatory studies are used, measuring and correlating all three provides the most comprehensive analysis of urethral competence.

The history and physical establish the diagnosis of SUI shed light on its severity and demonstrate the degree of urethral hypermobility. Urodynamics measures the leak point pressure, at what volume it occurs, and the severity of the leaking episodes.

Urodynamics is an art as much as a science, and the measurement of LPP is no exception. For example, a LPP of 20 cmH_2O is not a LPP of 140 cmH_2O in the same patient with SUI. It's established that significantly low LPP's are associated with lower surgical success rates, especially with trans-obturator or minimally invasive slings. In addition, a high leak point pressure in a women with mixed incontinence may signal to the provider that the overactive bladder is contributing more to the symptom complex, thereby influencing the diagnosis to treatment pathway.

During AUM, patients are instructed to perform activities that commonly reproduce their SUI, and to record the episodes using the event marker. This differentiates the stress leaks from other types of urinary incontinence. Investigators have used predefined stress activities as part of their ambulatory protocol, to help elicit SUI, and to reduce the number of false negatives.

In the urodynamics lab, the LPP is measured by instructing the patient to sequentially generate less powerful Valsalvas or coughs and recording it under direct supervision. Without adding a similar stress test to AUM, obtaining the lowest LPP will be challenging in the home setting.

Directly supervised stress tests will improve the accuracy of the ambulatory study. They may be done at various time points including immediately after insertion of the sensor, just before its removal, and at predetermined times, assuming that a portion of the study is performed in the clinic. It's helpful to determine the bladder volume with ultrasound prior to stress testing, as LPP's are commonly volume dependent.

An ecosystem could similarly assist in assessing urethral competence, and help paint the picture of the severity of the SUI and how it impacts the patient. Their recording of what they were doing at the time of the leak and the severity of the incontinence episode would be beneficial. A woman leaking a few drops only while playing tennis and needing a liner has less severe SUI, and is likely less impacted than one who uses three Depends per day and leaks large amounts while coughing, bending, walking, and during most activities.

Evaluation of voiding efficiency

Voiding efficiency can be evaluated by the history, physical, uroflowmetry, the post-void residual, and urodynamics. A combined approach represents the most thorough assessment.

During voiding, urodynamics evaluates the detrusor's ability to contract in a coordinated fashion and the urethra to relax simultaneously. Pressure flow is the gold standard in identifying the presence of poor bladder contractility and bladder outlet obstruction in patients with flow symptoms. The maximum voiding pressure, the Qmax generated, and whether or not the detrusor contraction is well sustained are important.

Assessing voiding efficiency with AUM has the potential of offering a number of advantages over conventional studies. Absence of the urethral catheter, elimination of the guarding reflex, physiologic filling not adversely affecting detrusor contractility, and providing a number of voids to assess may improve the evaluation. Learning how bladder volume affects voiding pressure, whether or not the patient normally strains to assist voiding, and an ecosystem that helps identify which voids best represent the patient symptoms will also be helpful.

Diagnostic to treatment pathways

As with conventional studies, I'm hopeful that AUM, when combined with a detailed history and physical examination and other testing will help providers establish the most effective diagnosis to treatment pathway in patients with lower urinary tract symptoms. I believe that both types of urodynamics, either used singly or in combination, will equip physicians to better counsel their patients, set realistic expectations, and troubleshoot when necessary. Providing excellent care for our LUTS patients is our ultimate goal.

Endnotes

1. Kobashi KC, Vasavada S, Bioschichak A, et al. Updates to surgical treatment of female stress urinary incontinence (SUI): AUA/SUFU guideline published (2017), amended (2023). J Urol. 2023; 209(6): 1091-1098.
2. Sandhu JS, Breyer B, Comiter C, et al. Incontinence after Prostate Treatment: AUA/SUFU Guideline (2019).
3. Sandhu JS, Bixler BR, Dahm P, et al. Management of lower urinary tract symptoms attributed to benign prostatic hyperplasia (BPH): AUA Guideline amendment 2023. J Urol. 2023; 10.1097/JU.0000000000003698
4. Lightner DJ, Gomelsky A, Souter L et al. Diagnosis and treatment of overactive bladder (non-neurogenic) in adults: AUA/SUFU Guideline amendment 2019. J Urol 2019; 202: 558.
5. Gormley EA, Lightner DJ, Burgio KL et al. Diagnosis and treatment of overactive bladder (non-neurogenic) in adults: AUA/SUFU Guideline. J Urol 2012; 188: 2455.
6. Clemens JQ, Erickson DR, Varela NP, Lai HH. Diagnosis and treatment of interstitial cystitis/bladder pain syndrome. J Urol. 2022; 208(1): 34-42.
7. Ginsberg DA, Boone TB, Cameron AP et al. The AUA/SUFU Guideline on Adult Neurogenic Lower Urinary Tract Dysfunction: Diagnosis and Evaluation. J Urol 2021; 206: 1097.
8. Ginsberg DA, Boone TB, Cameron AP et al: The AUA/SUFU Guideline on Adult Neurogenic Lower Urinary Tract Dysfunction: Diagnosis and Follow-up. J Urol 2021; 206: 1106.
9. Winters JC, Dmochowski RR, Goldman HB, et al. Adult Urodynamics: AUA/SUFU Guideline. J Urol. 2012
10. Davis DM. The Hydrodynamics of the upper urinary tract (urodynamics). Annals of Surg. 140: 839, 1954.
11. Gleason DM and Lattimer JK. The pressure-flow study: a method for measuring bladder neck resistance. J Urol. 87: 944, 1962.

12. Susset JG. Urodynamic society presidential address: Urodynamics- a step toward experimental urology. Neurourol and Urodynamics. 4:157-160, 1985.

13. Abrams P, Cardozo L, Fall M et al. The Standardization of Terminology of Lower Urinary Tract Function: Report from the Standardization Sub-committee of the International Continence Society. Neurourol and Urodynamics. 21: 167-178. 2002.

14. Bump RC, Mattiasson A, Bo K et al. The standardization of terminology of female pelvic organ prolapse and pelvic floor dysfunction. Am J Obstet Gynecol. 175: 10-17. 1996.

Acknowledgements

To David Staskin, MD

David, thank you for fine-tuning *The Art of LUTS* and letting me write in sometimes an unconventional manner. You have so many gifts to share with others. I love you like a brother. Cheers.

To Christine Nikas, MD

Thank you Christine for all of your edits. Your fabulous smile and wonderful mind are going to bless so many patients. Good luck in your career.

To Kari White

Kari, what can I say. You gave me your time, talent, and creativity and produced such a beautiful book. I will cherish your expertise and willingness to help me forever. God bless you.

To my friends at Laborie

Thank you for encouraging me to write this labor of love. Hopefully this book combined with your world-class equipment can help providers deliver excellence when treating patients with lower urinary tract dysfunction. Your steadfast commitment to urology and our sub-specialty is so appreciated.

I hope you enjoyed reading The Art of LUTS. Please don't hesitate to reread some of the sections, especially if you think that it would enhance your knowledge in caring for patients with lower urinary tract dysfunction. Remember to love your patients and good luck to you all.

Cheers.
Scott MacDiarmid, MD

ABOUT THE AUTHOR

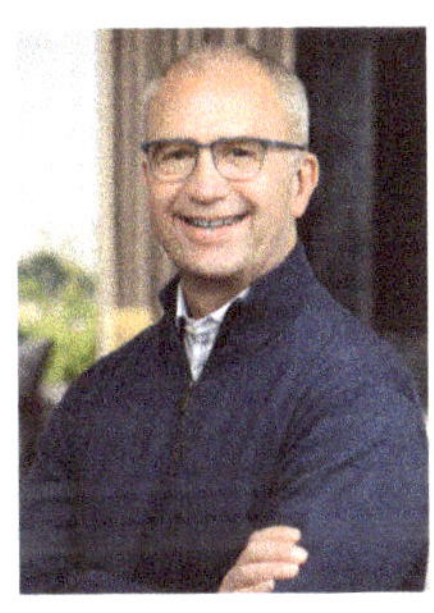 Dr. Scott MacDiarmid is deeply interested in and has given his career to helping patients with lower urinary tracts symptoms and pelvic floor disorders. Dr. MacDiarmid is director of the Alliance Urology Specialists Bladder Control Center in Greensboro, NC. He completed fellowships in reconstructive urology and urodynamics at Duke University Medical Center in Durham, NC; the University of Otago in Christchurch, New Zealand; and the University of Sheffield in England. He is currently an adjunct assistant professor of urology in the Department of Urology at the University of North Carolina in Chapel Hill, NC.